In Sickness

&

In Health

Caring for a Loved One with Alzheimer's

WILLIAM M. GRUBBS

ELDER BOOKS
Forest Knolls, California

Library of Congress Cataloging in Publication Data
Main Entry Under Title:
In Sickness & In Health: Caring for A Loved One With Alzheimer's
Grubbs, William.M.
1. Alzheimer's disease 2. Dementia 3. Caregivers 4. Nursing Homes

ISBN 0-943873-12-6
LCCN 94-061039
Printed in the United States of America

Cover & Book Design: Bonnie Fisk-Hayden

Dedications

To:

ACTO (Alzheimer's Caregivers Time Out), a volunteer day-care center where Bess found friends with whom she felt secure, gained a sense of belonging, and lost her feeling of social isolation; where she found recreational activities and lost her idleness, boredom, and frustrations; and where I found new friends, time out, and relief as a caregiver.

The Dunwoody and Decatur, Georgia, Alzheimer's family support groups, two lighthouses of help and hope, where I found new friends struggling with a similar tragedy; where we shared our experiences, our feelings, and even our humor without fear of being misunderstood; where I lost my sense of aloneness, found moral support, and gained an emotional lift from others coping with a common problem.

Jane L. Cope, former English and Latin teacher, who read, reread, and edited my writings and provided me friendship, conversation, and moral support.

Charles B. Pyles, PhD, friend and former colleague, who read and discussed each chapter and helped me keep alive interest in my former field of endeavor.

⌘

TABLE OF CONTENTS

A Personal Note

Most books about Alzheimer's have been written by professional health care people, such as a doctor or a nurse. I am neither a doctor nor a nurse, but a retired college professor. I write as a caregiver for my wife who died with Alzheimer's. I have told the story as it was, what it did to her, what it did to me, and what I did, as an elderly man, to save my own mental and emotional wellbeing during that long and terrible ordeal.

I have emphasized the importance of providing mental and social activities from which the patient can find a sense of meaning and pleasure as long as possible. Unfortunately, our traditional nursing homes are not well prepared to serve the needs of Alzheimer's patients and in the book, I emphasize that we need special places, special programs, and special attendants to care adequately for these unfortunate people. For the caregiver, I have emphasized the importance of social and emotional support which may be found in Alzheimer support groups, the importance of activities to preserve their own sanity, and the importance of humor.

It is my hope that all caregivers and all who may become caregivers, will find information, inspiration, and the moral support they need to survive that devastating disorder as well as I did.

William M. Grubbs

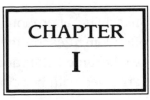

CHAPTER I

Meeting the Girl I Married

In late August, 1922, while a student in a junior college, a young lady came into a Latin class which I was attending. Since she was entering several days late, the friendly professor introduced her as Miss Bessie Tysinger. I had never heard the name before; the only thing that attracted my attention was her unusual last name. I do not recall speaking to her after class. Certainly, my later attraction to and relationship with her were not matters of "love at first sight."

It was not until Thanksgiving Day of the same year that we had an opportunity to meet and talk with each other. We were students at Mars Hill Junior College, a Baptist institution in North Carolina. Our football team was playing a game with the team of a nearby college, and except for a few dozen students, our campus was virtually empty.

It was a beautiful, sunny, November afternoon, and we boys, seeing the girls sitting on the front porch, walked over to spend the afternoon chatting while awaiting the return of the other students with news about the game. Since I knew her as a classmate, I joined Miss Tysinger. The only thing I remember from that conversation was the discovery that her home was in the same state as mine, North Carolina, and that we lived only about forty miles apart.

Following that Thanksgiving afternoon, we were on a first-name basis and we often joined each other at the dinner table in the dining hall. As we became better acquainted, I asked her for a date, which she arranged with her dormitory matron.

Courtship on a College Campus

Under the strict rules governing boy-girl relationships at the college, the same boy and girl were allowed only one date per month, and only on a Sunday afternoon. When a boy asked a girl for a date, she would get permission from her dormitory matron and, at two o'clock on Sunday afternoon, the boys gathered in front of the girls' dormitory to join their girlfriends. All the couples formed a line and, under the watchful eyes of the chaperones, we walked around the campus and into the rural area surrounding the college, often as much as two miles or more into the country and back. We called that arrangement the "soup line." I do not know why it was called the soup line for no soup, romantic or otherwise, was ever served in that line.

No touching or holding hands was permitted, and the girls suffered the penalties for any infractions of that rule by having their dating privileges denied. What a social revolution has occurred on the college campus since those days! Believe it or not, from that system of dating a number of happy marriages resulted.

I found Bess to be witty, fun-loving, friendly, intelligent, and good-looking, but tubby. Because she was overweight, A student had given her the nickname "Tubby," and "Tubby" she became to everyone. But, despite her extra avoirdupois, she was my kind of girl. After we married, she lost her nickname, but she remained tubby all her life.

In a student body of about 250, Bess knew everyone by name; I do not believe that any student had more friends nor more fun than she. Through it all, she maintained a high scholastic average. When I recently looked through her senior college yearbook, I found it filled with scribbled notes by both boys and girls, wishing her well and recalling funny incidents during their college days.

I can still recall a clandestine technique of courtship which made possible more frequent communication between two sweethearts. It was known by the unromantic title, the "city note", which was actually a love note enclosed in an envelope on which was written "city note." The notes were passed through trusted friends or, often, handed directly to the object of one's desire while going to class. Judging from what I read recently from a "city note" which Bess had stored away, such notes would make an interesting historical record on campus courtship during that era.

Through the "soup line," "city notes," table talk, train trips to our homes and back, and summer correspondence, Bess and I became better acquainted and discovered qualities in each other which we liked.

A Long and Happy Marriage

After five years of courtship, we had fallen in love and wanted to spend the rest of our lives together. We were married on December 24, 1927. I was twenty-six; she was twenty-four.

On our last wedding anniversary in 1990, we had been married 63 years, an unusually long marriage. The first unhappiness didn't occur until shortly before our 50th wedding anniversary, when I began to notice some puzzling symptoms in Bess which were later called "dementia."

I have been asked about the secrets of a happy marriage. I cannot speak about marriages in general, but I can suggest a number of factors which no doubt played a role in our happiness. Ours was not a case of "love at first sight," but was based on a five-year period of friendship and courtship. We were two mature people who had some understanding of ourselves and each other, and our marriage was based on that understanding, as well as love, loyalty, respect, patience, self-control, and humor. Bess and I believed that our marriage was a permanent partnership, which only death would end. Tolerance of and respect for each other's ideas and differences, as well as the ability to adjust, were essential ingredients.

I have always believed that Bess subscribed to the old motto that the nearest way to a man's heart is through his stomach. She was an excellent cook and this contributed much to my happiness and no doubt played a major role in our long and healthy lives. Humor also played an important role in our relationship. Bess was a collector of humorous plaques. She found one to express her feelings about the importance of cooking and hung it on the wall over the table in the breakfast room. It read: "Kissin' don't last. Good cookin' do." I must say, however, in our case, the "kissin'" did last. To defend herself against being overweight, she found a plaque which read: "A plump wife and a big barn never did any man harm." Still another read: "The opinions expressed by the husband in this house are not necessarily those of the management." Those plaques always hung on the wall where we could see them every day.

Not to be intimidated by her plaques, I found a few and hung them beside hers. One read: "Three things to hold in a marriage—your temper, your tongue, and each other." Another read: "The only way to fight a woman is with your hat. Grab it and run." Since I seldom wore a hat, if I saw trouble brewing, I was likely to grab my fly rod and head for the nearest trout stream, or the hoe, and start chopping in the garden. My neighbors might have accused me of killing snakes, but I was only working off my tensions.

Bess was a strong-willed, independent, and outspoken person with a quick wit and a sharp tongue, but never, prior to the onset of dementia, did she use that sharp tongue on me. There may have been times during our marriage when she felt like the wife whose friend asked her if she had ever thought of leaving her husband. The wife replied, "Shoot him, yes, but leave him, never." I, too, was strong-willed and independent-minded, but less witty and less sharp of tongue. We both hated quarreling and both had the ability to use self-restraint. Had this not been true, we might have had some angry brawls which would have left rifts in our marriage. Although we might disagree over where to place a rose bush or how to plant jonquil bulbs, we never disagreed seriously over the more fundamental things, like money, sex, politics, religion, or controversial public policies of our times.

Those are my views of our successful marriage. I would have liked to have Bess' views, but I never thought to ask until it was too late. I am sure that she would have agreed with me that we had a happy marriage. The years drew us closer together and we, in effect, became a part of each other. It hurt both of us very much when her dementia tore into our marriage.

Bess as the College and Local Community Knew Her

In college, Bess had majored in English Literature and, throughout her life, she retained that interest. She read many books and was an active member of a book club in the institution where I taught. She was always active in the social life of the faculty wives' clubs and played an important role in the social life of the community outside the college.

She had a great sense of humor and, despite dementia, that sense of humor survived. She loved to tell jokes, and was able to find humor in unexpected situations. Once, on her birthday, I took three cups of frozen ice cream to the nursing home and invited Bess and her friend, Mary, to share it with me. I said, "Mary, this is Bess' birthday. Do you think we should spank her?" Mary smiled, but before she could think of a response, Bess said, "It will take both of you to do that" and, in her typical style of finding a joke for every occasion, she told the following funny story: Little Johnnie had been very naughty and had so angered his mother that she turned him over her knees and spanked him vigorously with the palm of her hand. She then said, "Now, you go to your room and stay there for the afternoon." Little John went to his room, closed the door, pulled his pants down, turned his rear to the mirror and said, "Yep. Just as I thought. She busted it wide open."

In addition to being a wonderful wife and homemaker, Bess engaged in a number of outside activities which brought needed income to supplement that of a poorly paid college professor. Several times, she worked as a sales clerk in a department store, and she taught school for a short while. During World War II, she worked with the Red Cross, where her duties were to serve as intermediary between the men in the military service and their families back home. This required much driving alone over some of the most mountainous roads in the state, investigating, and reporting to the military. Because of these experiences, she had many interesting stories, which she enjoyed telling. After the War, she helped collect money for various forms of charitable relief. She served one term as president of the League of Women Voters in DeKalb County, and served on a local government commission to study and recommend reforms in the county government. For a number of years, she was in charge of a local voting precinct on election days. Since she had a great interest in local, state, and national politics, she worked in several campaigns, but never ran for political office. In her later years, she worked with the Red Cross Blood Mobile Units in our community.

Bess' most interesting and productive hobbies were weaving on an old-fashioned loom and creating pictures by needlecraft. On the loom, she made two beautiful bedspreads of virgin wool; with the needle she made beautiful pictures, many of which hung on the walls of our home and in the homes of our daughter and grandchildren. She was proud of her work and derived a great sense of achievement from it.

Forty Years in the Teaching Profession

Between 1927 and 1969, I spent 40 years in the teaching profession. Prior to World War II, salaries in that profession were very low and, despite some improvements after the war, it was not possible to become wealthy in the 40 years I spent teaching.

There were, however, other rewards — the satisfaction of having spent many years in a rewarding profession, and the feeling that I had made some contribution to the education of several thousand men and women. I also have pleasant memories of the students I taught and many unforgettable memories of the professional friendships and comradeship in a great and common cause. I had established the Department of Political Science at Georgia State University, had served as head of the department for 17 years, had risen to the rank of full professor, and had retired with the honorary title of Professor Emeritus. I have, however, one remaining greedy ambition — to live long enough to collect in teacher retirement what I think I should have been paid in salaries during my working years. Having already lived 24 years in retirement, I have made considerable progress toward that goal.

When I retired, I made an appraisal of our financial situation and discovered that, although by no means wealthy, we were

7

much better off than I had expected. We owned a comfortable home in a beautiful suburban area of Atlanta, and we had no debts. Our total income from teacher retirement, Social Security, and interest on our savings was enough to give us a sense of financial independence and security such as we had never felt before. Our two proudest financial achievements were our retirement income, which was above the average for retired couples, and our debt-free home. MediCare and insurance through the University System were sufficient to cover any major foreseeable medical and hospital bills.

As usual, Bess found a plaque which expressed her feelings about our achievements —- "We have done so much with so little for so long, we now think we can do anything at all with nothing in no time flat."

"The Golden Years of Our Old Age"

Someone, in a moment of wishful thinking, but with little experience with old age and none with Alzheimer's, coined the euphemistic term, "The Golden Years." It might have been more realistic to use the terms "The mixed blessings of old age" or "The bittersweet experience of old age."

For about eight years following my retirement, Bess and I enjoyed the good life and the sweetest things that can come to an aged couple. We could look back on a half- century of happily married life; we were in good health; we owned our home and were free of all debts; we were not rich, but we had a retirement income sufficient to provide a comfortable living and to do the traveling we had long wished to do. We felt financially independent. Moreover, we had time to devote to our hobbies, to do volunteer work with the Red Cross in our community and to enjoy our friends and family, including grandchildren and great-grandchildren. We could look forward to several years of happy, meaningful, and useful old age. Neither of us realized that a time bomb was ticking in Bess' brain which would destroy her memory and mental abilities, rob her of her personality, and plunge us into the bitterest tragedy that can befall any older couple. We have, indeed, had the bittersweet experience of old age. ✧

CHAPTER II

SIGNS OF A COMING TRAGEDY

About six years after retirement, I began to see incidents of strange behavior in Bess which I did not understand. She looked well; she was still very active; and her medical examinations did not uncover any problems. The things I saw were at first minor and infrequent, and they did not greatly disturb me. I cannot pinpoint the date on which I first saw such symptoms, nor can I say with any certainty which symptoms appeared first. I now know that Alzheimer's can be very insidious and difficult to recognize in its early stages. Our daughter and some of our friends saw the symptoms earlier than I. In my memory, one of the first indications of coming trouble was her tendency to become disoriented as to the day of the week and as to directions. If I went to mow the grass on a weekday, she might say, "Don't do that on Sunday." If, on a trip, we left the highway to get gas or to eat lunch, she would want to go in the wrong direction when we returned to the highway. I soon discovered that if she drove alone, she was likely to get lost.

Gradually, she began to lose her short-term memory. She would read a letter from a friend or a family member and, later in the day, insist that she had never seen the letter. One day we received a letter from the wife of an old friend telling us that her husband had died. I read it first, then handed it to Bess, saying "Gordon is dead." She read it and returned it to me without a word. When I started to reread it, she asked, "Who is the letter from?" In less than a minute, she had forgotten the letter so completely that she thought she had never seen it.

On an automobile trip, I discovered that she had lost her mathematical ability. We often made an odometer recording at the beginning of a trip and checked it against the reading at various points on the way. Once, while driving, I gave her the odometer reading and asked her to figure our mileage by subtracting the recording at the start of the trip. She could not do it.

Since early in our married life, we kept a joint checking account. This required that we keep accurate records in our respective checkbooks so that we would know our balance at the end of the month. One month, I discovered that she had kept no records.

There were other incidents, such as sudden and unusual outbursts of anger at me without any apparent reason, spells which disappeared as suddenly as they appeared. This was puzzling and contrary to her nature.

She made frequent criticisms of our daughter, accusing her of having taken something from our home without permission. She even accused Estelle of giving our house key to other people, so they could enter and take what they wanted. Not only did Bess accuse her of taking things from our home, but she tried to turn our grandchildren against their mother. During our long married life, I had never been extremely angry with Bess, nor had she ever been very angry with me. Now, her behavior threatened our good family relationships, and I could no longer restrain my feelings. I could see nothing wrong with her, nor any reason for what she was doing. For the first time, our marital happiness was breaking up, and I felt that it was her fault. She was becoming the kind of woman with whom I could not have lived, lest I come to hate her. What could I do? It did no good to try to talk her out of such behavior. I became so angry that I began to think of her as a shrew. That kind of anger was tearing my heart out and turning me into a different person. I had to find some way out of it.

We had a little summer cottage in a small resort area in North Carolina where we often spent weekends, or longer periods of time, during the summer. One Friday, when I had about reached my limit, I suggested that we go to the mountains for a few days, and she agreed. When we arrived, we discovered that two good friends from Ohio, with a cottage near ours, were already there. The four of us got together that night and had a delightful time talking and playing an old game called "Aggravation." The next day, Chuck and I went fishing while Bess and Martia spent time together. Friends, fun, and fishing did wonders for me.

Since Bess was happy there, and an entirely different person from what she had been, I thought of another possible solution to our problem. Why not sell our home and move to a retirement home far away from our daughter and the grandchildren? That, to me, was a terrible thought, but it might be better than what we were experiencing. We visited a number of retirement communities, but I could never find one to which I could commit myself. They were not the kinds of places where I could spend the rest of my life, and I did not think that Bess, in the long run, would enjoy such a life either. I enjoyed occasional fishing, but I had to have something more meaningful in my life than playing golf, tennis, and other games. I now know that such a move would have been a terrible mistake.

It was about this time that Bess began, without explanation, to withdraw from her outside activities —the bridge club, the book club, and volunteer work with the Red Cross. She also gave up her position as manager of the voting precinct on election days. She began to lose interest in her most beloved hobby, needlecraft, but she kept buying new patterns, some of which were never finished.

Over the years since I first became aware of the onset of her dementia, I have recalled a number of things she did and said which were puzzling at that time, but now seem significant. One of her most pleasurable and meaningful activities, her hobby of making pictures with the needle and thread, was the last to go. As that skill declined, she seemed to work vigorously to finish more pictures. She began to tell a little story to me, to our daughter, and to the grandchildren. I heard her tell it many times, and it was very unusual for her. It was the story of a grandmother who made pictures with the needle and thread. She gave her most beautiful one to her granddaughter. Many years later, after the grandmother had died, the granddaughter suddenly discovered the monetary value of the picture when she was in need of surgery, which she could not afford. She offered the picture for sale, and the price she received helped pay the medical bill. Why did she repeatedly tell that story? She may have been aware of her declining skill and was seeking some sense of worth or achievement. She continued to buy new patterns, including the canvas and the thread, which she would start, but never finish.

Bess was once a great conversationalist, but with the onset of dementia, she lost her ability to converse about anything. Soon, conversation became a lost art in our lives, and that is not good for a marriage. Our inability to talk to each other about our lives, about what was going on around us, and about what was happening to her, led to boredom and frustration. Life became more and more dull and meaningless for both of us..

These incidents both puzzled and worried me. What was most confusing was the fact that Bess still looked well, not at all sick. Neighbors or friends who came to visit, hardly noticed

14

anything wrong with her. The only thing that might be noticed was that she did not take her usual part in the conversation. When I took her to the doctor, he could not see the symptoms which I was noticing. Usually, she seemed perfectly normal. I could not talk to a neighbor or a friend about her since none of them could see anything wrong. They might think I was losing my mind. It was becoming increasingly clear that I was living with a changing person; she was not the same Bess whom I had known and lived with so many years. I did not yet realize that we were facing the greatest tragedy of our lives, nor did I know that Bess was not responsible for what she was saying and doing. ↔

CHAPTER III

A SHOCKING DISCOVERY:
DEMENTIA OF THE ALZHEIMER TYPE

Because of my deep concern about what was happening to Bess, I arranged to take her to her doctor about two months earlier than her scheduled visit. When she came out of the examination room, she seemed agitated and ill at ease, and there were tears in her eyes; however, I said nothing until we were on our way home. Finally I asked, "How did you get along today?" She replied, "He didn't do anything." That surprised me, for she had been in his office the usual time for such examinations. I asked, "What do you mean?" She repeated that he had not done anything. I then asked about the EKG, the X-ray, and blood tests. Her response to every question was negative, but after a few minutes she said, "Maybe he did do the blood tests." I was sure that he had put her through the regular routine, but that she had forgotten and that she was terribly confused.

I have always wondered what happened in the doctor's office that day to cause her to come out so agitated. Did the doctor "blow his top" over something she did? He had been her doctor for more than twenty years, and it was very strange that she came out of his office in that condition. Since she absolutely refused to see that doctor again, I had to find another. Because she was in the early stages of Alzheimer's, I could not be sure that anything out of the ordinary had happened to produce in her such a state of confusion.

When we arrived home, I called the doctor's office and arranged an appointment to see him the next day. I told him what had happened and when I asked about the examination, he said he had done all the usual tests. It was then that he told me her problem was senile dementia, but he did not mention Alzheimer's. He offered to arrange a brain scan, and I agreed to have one scheduled as soon as possible.

When I returned home, Bess asked where I had been and, when I told her, she flew into an angry rage. I had never seen her so angry. She denounced me for going to the doctor without her and threatened to kill me and commit suicide. That was the only time she ever threatened me personally with bodily harm, but later she told our daughter that she was going to run a butcher knife through me. Although I had a shotgun which she knew how to use, I did not believe she would use either it or a knife. To be safe, however, I removed the gun, but not the knife, since I felt more able to defend myself from a knife than from a gun.

The brain scan was given a few days later. It is called a CAT scan, an acronym for Computerized Axial Tomography. The scan helps determine the presence of tumors, blood clots, hemorrhages, brain injuries, and strokes, but it cannot identify certain physical characteristics in the brain which are the distinguishing features of Alzheimer's disease. A CAT scan may not be able to determine evidence of very small strokes which, in large numbers, may cause Alzheimer-like symptoms. I was thankful the CAT scan did not show any of the above, but it left a lot of questions unanswered.

Some Confusion In Terminology

Until about two decades ago, most doctors were using the

terms "senile" and "hardening of the arteries" to define what was happening to older people in whom they found what are now called "Alzheimer-type symptoms." Some still use those terms. When doctors began to use the term "Alzheimer's Disease," there followed a period of confusion in terminology. Terms ranged from "senile dementia" to "pre-senile dementia" to "dementia of the Alzheimer type" and "chronic brain syndrome," to define symptoms which often were indistinguishable.

The words "senile" and "dementia" had frightening connotations. To me, "senile" meant loss of memory, confusion, and disorientation associated with extreme old age, and I had known very few people who were senile. It was difficult for me to think of Bess as being old and senile; she did not look old, nor did she act old, except for her minor dementia symptoms. "Dementia," for me, had the connotation of "crazy" or "insane." Did senile dementia mean that she was both senile and crazy? I wanted some clarification of terminology and some answers.

After much reading and research, I discovered that doctors do not use dementia to define a disease, but rather to denote a group of symptoms, such as loss of memory, confusion, disorientation, and decline of intellectual ability. These symptoms are caused either by a disease or diseases in the brain itself, or by some condition or disorder in the body which may affect the brain. Since it is impossible to make a definitive diagnosis prior to autopsy, many doctors began to use the terms Dementia of the Alzheimer Type, (DAT); Senile Dementia of the Alzheimer's Type, (SDAT); and Alzheimer's Disease, (AD).

I have been deeply concerned about the possibility that Bess may have inherited Alzheimer's. If this is true, it is possible that she and I have unknowingly passed a faulty gene, or genes, to our daughter and to our grandchildren. She had two sisters who died after a period of similar symptoms, although neither was diagnosed as having Alzheimer's. She lost a brother to Parkinson's Disease and a second cousin to Down's Syndrome. It has been well-established that there is a familial problem in about 10% of cases, but most people who have Alzheimer's have no record of it in their families. Although there have been a number of research efforts in this area, it has not been possible to establish any definitive conclusions as to the risk incurred by one who has family members with Alzheimer's. Some scientists think the risk may depend upon the closeness of the relationship, the number of family members with Alzheimer's, and the age of onset. Many believe that there may be more than one type of familial Alzheimer's—early onset and late onset. Why does the risk of contracting the disease increase with age? Could it be that faulty genes lie dormant in most or all of us, but for some reason do not become activated until late in life? If this is true, and if we could find a way to delay or suppress the activating factor for five or ten years, we might save many people from the horrors of Alzheimer's.

I get some comfort from Howard Gruetzner's statement: "The idea that Alzheimer's can run in families leads many relatives of Alzheimer's victims to wonder whether they, too, will someday fall prey to the disease. In the great majority of cases, the answer is No. For most close relatives of an Alzheimer's victim, the statistical risk of getting the disease is just slightly greater than for the general population. The only persons with a real basis for concern are those whose families have documented cases of early-onset Alzheimer's and cases in preceding generations, and those who have more than one first-degree relative affected in the current generation." [1]

[1] Howard Gruetzner, Alzheimer's, *A Caregiver's Guide And Source Book,* John Wiley and Sons, Inc., New York, 1988, p. 48.

Gene Therapy: The Ultimate Technique of Medicine

Since Bess and two of her sisters had died with Alzheimer's-type symptoms, my desire to know more about genetics was aroused. There is no way to know with any certainty that Bess' problem was genetic in nature; but the possibility that it was propelled me to learn more about the gene, and the scientific breakthroughs made in recent years relative to it. Those scientific developments have made possible the use of a new medical technique which, if successful, may be the most revolutionary achievement in medical science in 2,000 years. Gene therapy—the ability to restructure the human gene to cure or to prevent genetic diseases—has been called by some "the ultimate medicine." To work with the essence of life itself, to play God with human life—this development is so important that average people need to know about it and the problems it raises.

Let us begin with the cell, the smallest living component of the human body. No one knows how many cells there are in the body, but it is agreed that there are trillions. Each cell has a nucleus, which is the heart and control center of the cell. Each normal cell has 46 thin, threadlike structures called "chromosomes." Within the chromosomes are 50,000 to 100,000 genes. The chromosomes and genes are made up of the DNA (deoxyribonucleic acid). Since the genes pass hereditary materials from one generation to the next, it is important that we understand their nature and functions.

The cells of a man's body create millions of sperm in the testes. The cells of a woman's body create eggs in her ovaries. Somehow, the cells of their bodies know to include in each sperm and each egg only 23 chromosomes, just half the number 46 of a normal cell, the beginning of a new human being. Through this unique process, the new cell gets half its chromosomes and genes from the father and half from the mother. Immediately after conception, this new cell begins to divide and multiply, creating more cells. Each normal cell contains all the 46 chromosomes and all the genes of the original cell. Each cell thus carries the hereditary materials from both the father and the mother and is able to multiply and reproduce itself. Each cell has the capacity to form any organ in the body and to perform the functions of that organ — the heart, the liver, the kidneys, the brain, the eyes, and so on. Each gene carries the physical characteristics and features of both the father and the mother, such as color of the eyes, the color of the hair, the size of the nose, and one's general appearance. We often say that the daughter or the son favors one or the other of the parents, or that he or she has certain features of one parent or the other. Each cell also carries both the good genes and the bad genes from both the father and the mother to the newborn son or daughter.

Through a process of differentiation, a division of labor, the cells multiply, group, and specialize to form certain organs and to perform certain functions of the body. Although each cell has the capacity to form any of those organs and perform their functions, they group and use only a part of their potential to form one certain organ, such as the heart, the kidneys, the lungs, the eyes, the brain, and so on. Somehow, they know when to start the process, when to stop it, and where to place each organ. This miracle, we do not understand.

As unbelievable as it may seem, there is a ceaseless and never-ending process within each cell. That process consists of converting the food we eat into energy and manufacturing the proteins and chemicals essential to our bodily activities. In essence, there is a chemical manufacturing plant within each of those microscopic components of our body.

In recognition of the profound importance of deciphering the human gene for both medical science and mankind in general, scientists and governments are undertaking what has been called by some "the gene hunt" and by others "mapping the human genome." These efforts are underway in Japan, England, Italy, West Germany, France, and the U.S. In January, 1989, at the National Institutes of Health (NIH) in Washington, the Human Genome Advisory Committee launched a program called the Human Genome Project. Its purpose is to map the human genome, which may rival both the Manhattan Project (which built the atom bomb) and the Apollo moon-landing program (which landed a man on the moon). Some scientists think it may eventually exceed both in importance. The effort is estimated to cost $3 billion, and it is hoped that it will be completed in 20 years. The U.S. government is providing the funds.

The goal is to locate, map and analyze every one of the 100,000 human genes that shape a human being, from embryo to adult, to decipher the secrets of the gene. The gene, which contains a complete set of instructions for making a human being, is tucked away in the nucleus of each of the trillions of cells in the human body. Encoded in the DNA of the infant's 46 chromosomes are instructions that affect not only structure, size, coloring and other physical attributes, but also intelligence, susceptibility to disease, and even some aspects of behavior. The ultimate goal of the Human Genome Project is to read and understand these instructions. If successful, it will enable us to understand the very essence of our lives. Dr. James Watson, who heads up the project, says, "I see an extraordinary potential for human betterment ahead of us... We can have at our disposal the ultimate tool for understanding ourselves. The time to act is now." [2]

The achievement of the goal would enable doctors to identify

[2] Atlanta Constitution.

the causes of thousands of genetic disorders. It would be possible to predict the vulnerability of an individual to hereditary diseases and to prescribe drugs or alter the genome to prevent it.

If and when we have unraveled the mysteries of the brain and can read the messages in our genes, we will not yet be "out of the woods." Such achievements will indeed be a long step forward in our search for the cause and cure of Alzheimer's and other diseases, and give us hope, but that hope is likely to be long-term. Once we understand the cause, or causes, we must find the cures.

It may require 20 years to complete the gene-mapping project but, if successful, it will make it possible to prepare a genetic profile of an individual—to locate bad genes, as well as the absence of the normal genes essential to the proper functioning of the immune system. If experiments in gene therapy are successful, it will be possible to depress or remove the bad genes and replace them with normal genes, or good genes, from another human being. The profile could reveal what diseases we are more susceptible to. Although this kind of information would make it possible for us to prevent or prepare for diseases for which we are at risk, it could also make one unemployable and uninsurable.

For the first time in late 1990, the Food and Drug Administration gave the green light to a group of doctors to try gene therapy on a human being. The patient was an unidentified four-year-old child who was suffering from adenosine deaminase deficiency (ADA). ADA is a very rare immune system disorder, which is incurable and deadly. It was this disorder which killed David, the "Bubble Boy." The child lacked a normal gene essential for the functioning of her immune system. The doctors took a normal gene from another person, placed it in a white blood cell of the child, and then injected that into her to help start her immune system to work.

Let us suppose that the gene-mapping program is eventually completed, and that it becomes possible to make a genetic profile of an individual. Think for a moment about the problems which might arise. Would you want a genetic profile of yourself? Would you permit a prospective employer to see that profile? Would you permit an insurance agent to see it? Would you wish to see the genetic profile of the person you wished to marry? Would you permit the prospective bride or groom to see your profile? The down side of genetic profiling is that it would open the door to a new type of discrimination.

How far should gene therapy go? Should it be used for any purpose other than curing genetic diseases? Suppose it became possible, through genetic engineering and therapy, to influence the features of a fetus in the process of development in the womb; i.e., to make a baby "to order." A couple might give instructions for a baby with blue eyes, brown hair, the physique of a football player, the talent of an artist or a musician. One may laugh at such suggestions, but if gene therapy really works, it will be possible to play God with the very essence of life. What are we going to do with that power? I have seen many undreamed-of things happen during my life, and the age of miracles is far from being over.

It is time for the general public—those of us who are not scientists—to begin to think about this "ultimate medicine" and to ponder the ethical problems which may be involved. Although it has a great potential for both good and bad, there is no turning back now. ✎

CHAPTER
IV

THE IMPACT OF ALZHEIMER'S DISEASE

Alzheimer's disease has a devastating emotional, mental, and physical effect on the victim and the family, particularly on the caregiver who is most often a wife, a husband, or a daughter. Without a successful coping program and moral support from others, the caregiver is in danger of becoming a secondary victim of the disease. In an effort to describe the impact of the disease, caregivers have used a number of terms: "a living death," "an unending funeral," "another name for insanity," "a living hell." I have experienced a few moments of each and will add one more to that list: "The ultimate tragedy of old age." There are, of course, other dementias and chronic diseases which can be terrible tragedies, but I believe none can compare in suffering and cruelty with Alzheimer's. The disease has been for me like a Greek tragedy, in that I knew very early what the ultimate end would be, the death of Bess' mind, but I was fated to watch its inexorable progress to the bitter end. That was indeed a "living death" and an unending grief from which there was no relief until Bess' physical death.

The Cruel Impact of Alzheimer's on Bess

Before the onset of dementia, Bess was intelligent, independent, outspoken, humorous, and sociable. She enjoyed her life and relationships, and found meaning, purpose, and a sense of achievement in her activities and hobbies. With the onset of Alzheimer's, she ceased to be the person she used to be. She lost her memory, her self-initiative, her self-control, and her ability to think. The loss of such vital human qualities had a devastating impact on her. She was no longer able to engage in a social relationship and she felt socially isolated. She could no longer remember the names of people. Since she could no longer read, watch TV, or carry on a conversation, she was reduced to a state of idleness, boredom, confusion, and helplessness. She no longer felt secure, except at home and in my presence.

Despite all those losses, she was still very much alive and human, and she still had certain desires and needs. Moreover, she retained certain physical and mental abilities but having lost her self-initiative and know-how, she could not, without help, use them to satisfy her desires and needs. I cannot imagine a worse hell-on-earth than to be reduced to such a state. She was still able to suffer emotionally and mentally. She needed tender loving care and the human touch to help her find meaning in activities and friendly social relationships. Without help, life for her became meaningless and she became tired of living.

The Impact on Me as Husband and Caregiver

I am, by nature, a compassionate and empathetic person, but I had never imagined that one could suffer so many mixed emotions – guilt, grief, anger, frustration, helplessness, and hopelessness. Bess' condition and her suffering put me through hell on earth. My grief became chronic and left me only when I could keep my mind off what was happening to her and the suffering she was experiencing. The only relief I could find was in reading, writing, or working in the garden. I was told by some that, since I had done all I could for her, I should cease to feel guilt, but I was never able to rid myself completely of that feeling. I was deeply disappointed that, because of Alzheimer's, we were losing so many years of happy and useful life in our old age. One great disappointment was the absence of a nursing home or other facility which had the staff and the facilities to meet her special needs. I could see in Bess some surviving capabilities which could have been used by a skilled staff to meet her needs. I could not do it myself but, if I could have found such an institution, it would have relieved me of my major emotional and mental burdens. I could not help feeling that the doctors, the nurses, and the general public are not fully aware of what we are doing to many of the unfortunate victims of Alzheimer's. When placed in a nursing home, these people are simply housed in an institution lacking a staff to provide the activities and social contacts they really need. This feeling was a source of great frustration and suffering for me. It is my hope that, with growing awareness, our moral ethics and our caring natures will compel us to find ways to help these people to have a better life for as long as possible.

Being an inveterate dreamer, I cannot remember awaking without having had a dream or being in a dream. For the most part, my dreams have been pleasant, or at least not frightening nightmares. While Bess was in a nursing home, however, I frequently had a nightmare in which I found myself in a helpless, and often frightening, situation. One night in my dream, I was at the end of a narrow, steep, crooked mountain road, without knowing how I had arrived there, nor where I was going. There was no way to go forward, no way to turn around, and no way to go back. I was alone in a place I had never seen before, with a sensation of utter confusion and helplessness.

On another night, I dreamed that I had come to a city with

which I was familiar and had registered in a hotel where I had been before. After dinner I took a walk down a familiar street and, at the end of my walk, I turned and walked back on the same street to the hotel. When I arrived at the point where the hotel was supposed to be, there was no hotel. No one I asked could remember that there had ever been such a hotel in the city. I felt utterly confused and lost.

The most frightening dream occurred when I found myself sitting on the very edge of a steep cliff, with both feet hanging over the cliff and not a shrub or even a clump of grass within reach. I was afraid to move lest I slip off into what appeared to be a canyon several hundred feet deep. There was no one else in sight and I was completely helpless.

In the nursing home I often saw Bess and her roommate behaving like two little sisters quarreling over an article of clothing. These scenes finally caused a dream with a deep and lasting emotional effect on me. In that dream, I saw her in the body of an 85-year-old woman, acting like a little child taking its first steps. She came toward me, unsteady on her feet, mouth and eyes open, hands outstretched, reaching to me, and trying to get to me before she fell. That was a vivid picture of the condition to which Alzheimer's had reduced her, and I will never forget it. How does one cope with such a dream?

What produced such dreams? What significance, if any, did they have? Did they come from my frustrations and helpless feelings about Bess, or were they the ticking of an Alzheimer's bomb in my brain?

It is a well-known fact that, as we grow older, we become more vulnerable to Alzheimer's disease. Until a few months ago, I could take a positive attitude toward that risk. It was estimated that, for those of us who are 85 or older, the risk of succumbing to that dreaded disease was 25 percent, or about one out of four. I could then say that my chances were three out of four of escaping that fate. According to a new study of those risks, my chances are now estimated to be 47 percent, about one-out-of-two. I no longer have any basis for a positive attitude, and I can only hope that I may be the fortunate one of the two who escapes that cruel fate.

I am reminded of the legend of Damocles, a royal courtier of ancient Syracuse. In order to teach him a lesson about the perils of a ruler's life, he was seated at a feast table, with a sword hanging directly over his head, which was held by a single hair. That legend should teach those of us over 85 something of the perils of growing old. The sword of Alzheimer's hangs over our heads, held by a single gray hair, and the possibility of its dropping increases with every passing hour.

Despite the impact on me of what has happened to Bess, despite my old age and the threat that hangs over my head as I grow older, I still love life, and I still have the will to live. Frankly, I have never worried about my risks of developing Alzheimer's. Although my memory is poor, I see no loss of memory indicative of Alzheimer's.

A Second Victim of Alzheimer's Came Under my Care

Bess had three sisters, two of whom died with Alzheimer's-type symptoms. Both died before Bess did, and there was no autopsy performed on the brain of either. Although we have no proof other than their symptoms, I believe that both sisters may have had the same disease as Bess, and that she may have inherited the disease from her family.

When Bess and I moved to Atlanta, her sister Mamie had been living there for 15 years or more. She had never been married, never owned a home, nor had she owned or driven a car. She had lived alone and depended on the streetcar or bus for transportation. She and Bess had always had a good sisterly relationship, but they saw each other infrequently. Bess, being the older of the two, had always felt protective of Mamie. Our move to Atlanta provided an opportunity for them to renew their family relationship, which they quickly did.

When Mamie retired at age 65, we asked her to move to an apartment near our home so that she and Bess might see each other more often, and we could take her with us to the grocery store each week. Following the buying of our groceries, we always invited Mamie home for lunch. Since both of them were humorous and enjoyed reminiscing about their early family life, I enjoyed listening and learning more about their family than I had ever known before.

Four or five years after Mamie moved near our home, I began to notice some strange symptoms in her. Since she loved cats, she often took strays into her apartment as pets. This was not strange or unusual and did not concern me because I knew pets provided some relief in her lonely life. Soon, however, I noticed her bill for cat food was almost equal to her own grocery bill, and she began to spend more time discussing her cats and their behavior than any other subject of conversation.

A few months later, when she came home with us for lunch, she complained that the man who lived in the apartment underneath her had rigged the electrical wiring so that she was paying not only her bill, but his also. Although I doubted that claim, I promised to check into it when we returned home after lunch. As I expected, her suspicions were unfounded. My explanations did not satisfy her, and she continued to believe that she was paying his electric bill, as well as her own. Since July had been an exceptionally hot month and electric bills were soaring to new heights, I assumed that her unusually high bills, plus the fact that she did not understand the electrical wiring system, were responsible for her misunderstanding.

A few months later, however, I discovered a more serious symptom of a mental problem. Mamie called and asked, "Bill, do you know anyone who would buy my furniture?" That amazed me, and I asked what was wrong and why she wished to sell her furniture. She said, "They have stopped my Social Security checks, and I cannot pay my bills." I was so astonished I didn't argue with her. I simply said, "Mamie, just hold everything until I can get there."

When Bess and I arrived, we found her visibly confused and agitated. When I tried to talk with her for a few minutes, I discovered that she could give me no sensible answer to anything I asked. I then asked to see her checkbook. When I saw it, I could not "make heads nor tails" of it. There were the names of the utility company and the apartment house where she lived, but no amount of any check she had written. In some cases, the amount of a check was written where the number should have been, and the number where the amount should have been. As I looked over the records in her checkbook, I could not tell what her balance was, if any. I knew then that she had a mental problem and could no longer manage her finances. Since Bess was already suffering from Alzheimer's, I thought to myself, "Oh, my God! Do I have another person under my care who is losing her mind?"

After looking at her check book, I said, "Let's go to the bank." There I discovered that she had already paid her bills for that month and still had enough in her account to pay the bills for the next month. Her Social Security checks had not stopped coming to the bank, but I discovered that unless she found a cheaper apartment and got rid of the cats, she would exhaust her bank account within a few months. She was living beyond her income.

Since there was no other person in her family who could assume the responsibility of managing her finances, I asked that we withdraw the remainder of her account and establish a joint account with my bank. From that time onwards, I held the checkbook, wrote all checks, and gave her a weekly cash allowance. I continued this arrangement until she reached the point where she could no longer be trusted with cash to pay her grocery bill.

My next problem was to find her an affordable apartment. I turned to the apartments for the elderly, which were subsidized by HUD. All were full and had long waiting lists. When I discovered, however, another apartment house which was in the process of being built, I hastened to the agency in charge. Although not yet completed, the management still had vacancies and was accepting applications. Since it was supposed to be ready for occupancy within two months, I assumed the responsibility as her sponsor and rented an apartment on the spot. Her rent and utility bills would be a certain percentage of her income, thus saving $145.00 per month. It was farther away from our home and much more inconvenient, but it was the best I could find.

It was at this point that my daughter, Estelle, came to my assistance and made arrangements for Mamie's move. She also assumed the responsibility of looking after Mamie's clothing and seeing that she took baths frequently. For awhile, I continued giving Mamie a weekly cash allowance for groceries. Her new residence was a long distance from both Estelle and me, and as her mental condition deteriorated, each of us was making two or three trips every week. Bess continued to go with me until I had to put her in a nursing home, although the two could no longer engage in conversation.

At first, Mamie seemed happy in her new home. She made new friends, and soon forgot the cats. Her mental condition, however, continued to deteriorate more rapidly than had been true with Bess. Within about 18 months, she could no longer buy groceries, and I had to take on that responsibility. She had stocked her shelves, refrigerator, and freezer full of canned meats, vegetables, and fruits, which she was not eating. Soon, she could neither cook her own meals nor even heat water for coffee. We applied to Meals-on-Wheels to bring one hot meal a day, five days a week. For the other meals, Estelle and I took her ready-cooked food.

The Impact of Alzheimer's on Estelle

When Mamie developed Alzheimer's disease, Estelle came to my rescue and largely assumed the responsibility of caring for her until we placed her in a nursing home. Without Estelle's help, I would have had two demented persons on my hands. Although I had wanted both a son and a daughter, since we had only one child, I was now thankful it had been a daughter.

To know that her mother and her two aunts were all victims of the same cruel disease was a shocking experience for Estelle. Although she fears that she herself may become a victim through inheritance, she has been able to cope very well with that burden. Like her mother, she is energetic and active and finds relief from her forebodings in activities and in social relationships. She has become an accomplished tole painter, painting on fabric, wood, and metal, and spends every spare moment painting. She also finds a ready market for her work. This gives her a sense of worth and achievement and keeps her mind off her problems. She and her friends who are engaged in the same hobby often meet and spend the day together painting. She has also found a part-time job with a publishing company. Her painting and her social relationships have been her coping techniques and her source of achievement. ❧

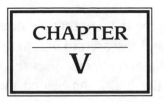

CHAPTER
V

WHEN THE BRAIN,
"THE DIVINIST PART OF US," FAILS

Why Study the Brain?

Although the primary purpose of my education was to develop, improve, and learn how to use the potential capacities of my brain, my textbooks or teachers never said much about that miraculous organ. Even though I made my livelihood by using my brain, I never thought or read much about that "divinest part" of me. It was not until I discovered what was happening to Bess and learned that the source of her problem was the brain that I developed an interest in making a special study of that organ and how it functions. The more I learned about it, the more convinced I became that it is, indeed, not only the "divinest part," but also the most complex and important organ in the body. Those are sufficient reasons for getting better acquainted with the brain.

Since Bess' dementia symptoms were caused by what was happening in her brain, my curiosity was aroused to know more about how that organ functions. This I needed to know if I were to understand her condition, cope with it successfully, and care for her. It would help me to place the blame for her behavior where it *belonged*, and *not on her.*

It has given me hope to learn that the brain is now the subject of intensive study and research to unfold its mysteries, to find a means of diagnosing Alzheimer's disease, and to devise a cure. My knowledge of the brain has helped me to understand the nature and complexity of that search, and what I have learned has given me new hope that a cure will be found.

My study of the brain has not only satisfied my curiosity, but has proved to be an effective coping device and good therapy.

The Nature and Functions of the Brain

Plato, the Greek philosopher, said of the brain, "It is the divinest part of us and the Lord of all the rest." The legendary founder of medicine, Hippocrates, said, "Not only our pleasures, our joy and laughter, but also our sorrow, pain, grief, and tears arise from the brain, and the brain alone. With it, we think and understand, we see and hear, and we discriminate between the ugly and the beautiful, between what is pleasant and what is unpleasant, and between good and evil." [3]

"We don't just use or depend on our brains, we are our brains. Everything we feel, say, think, or do comes from the brain. We cannot take a breath, or wake up, without directions from these three pounds of soft, wet, pinkish gray tissue ... an unprepossessing mass which somehow manages to hold all our memories, our understanding of the world, our dreams." [4]

"Language and abstract thought, judgment, planning, advanced reasoning, and learning—all of these would be impossible without the highly developed human brain. But the brain is much, much more than the center of intellectual activity. You need your brain to breathe, to metabolize food, and even to excrete wastes. The brain regulates and coordinates all volun-

[3] Tolstar Books, *The Brain: Mystery of Mind and Matter*, New York, 1984, p. 9.
[4] National Geographic Society, *The Incredible Machine*. New York, 1984, p. 9.

tary and involuntary moves, all sensory impressions, and all the emotions. Without your brain, you could not appreciate a painting or a poem, a symphony or a scenic vista. To your brain, you owe your consciousness of yourself and the world around you, your unconscious life, your creativity, your personality." [5]

All animals and birds have brains, but our brain is different. It has capacities which make us human and different from all other animals. We can learn, remember, think, reason, plan, visualize, make tools and machines, perceive and solve problems, develop languages and writing, find the causes of diseases in our bodies, and devise cures or means of prevention, create sciences, and perform miracles. The human brain has an unlimited potential for improvement and development. Every human being who is capable of doing so should have some appreciation of that miraculous organ in the top of his head. For the first time in history, we are developing techniques for seeing the live human brain in action. If the brain can devise such techniques, can we use those products of our brain to better understand and find cures for all the diseases and conditions which are causing the Alzheimer's-type symptoms in that organ? The brain and the human gene hold the very essence of life itself. If we can unravel and use their mysteries, we will have the power to transform life itself. That would be the ultimate medicine. What will we do with it? Surely we can find a cure for Alzheimer's. I quote the neuroscientist Francis O. Schmitt, "Whether one likes it or not, man has embarked on the greatest of human experiences ... that of determining whether ... man can discover the mechanism of thinking, and whether, by so doing, he can achieve a new order of understanding ... the dimensions of his own nature." [6]

[5] *Reader's Digest*, ABC's Of The Human Body. 1987, p. 46.
[6] Tolstar Books, *The Brain: Mystery Of Mind And Matter.* p. 151

The Geography of the Brain

On top of the head, just under the skull, are the right and left hemispheres of the brain. They are very much alike in form and appearance. We have two brains, a matched pair, and each has the capacity to act independently of the other, but they are not necessarily equal. The left brain controls certain actions and features of the right side of the body. Most people are right-handed; that explains why, in most people, the left hemisphere of the brain is larger than the right. Each hemisphere specializes in controlling certain human functions. The left brain controls reading, writing, mathematics, reasoning, and scientific skills; and the right brain specializes in controlling art awareness, musical awareness, imagination, and insight. A group of nerve fibers, called the corpus callosum, connects the two brains and enables them to operate as a coordinated whole.

The outer surface of the brain is called the cerebral cortex. It contains 75% of the estimated 100 billion nerve cells, or neurons, in the brain. There, in a nut shell, is where we find those parts of the brain whose functions serve to make us human. Other areas are important, but these are the locations of the tangles and plaques, which are the distinguishing features of Alzheimer's, and they are parts which, if impaired, produce the Alzheimer symptoms. These are the parts of the brain that store our memories, evoke our imagination, produce our language, and control our motivations, our self-reliance, our personality, and our behavior.

We have quite a way to go yet before we can be too specific about the function of each part of the brain and before we can understand their interrelationships, but they seem to be the parts that have most to do with such human characteristics as memory, emotions, thinking, personality, and behavior. If the nerve cells or neurons are dead or impaired in these areas, or their communications with each other are disrupted, Alzheimer-type symptoms will result. These are the areas where intensive research is underway to determine what is happening and why. Are the neurons dead or dying? If so, why? Is there a breakdown in the intercommunications, the transfer of messages from one neuron to another? If so, why? Much emphasis is now centered on the latter.

Each hemisphere of the brain is divided into four lobes. These are the frontal lobes, the parietal lobe, the temporal lobe, and the occipital lobe. The frontal lobes have something to do with motor functions, emotional behavior, personality, and social behavior. The parietal lobe is related to sensory functions and is called the "feeling" part of the brain. The temporal lobe is concerned with hearing, memory, sense of self and, perhaps, our emotions. The occipital lobe is the vision center of the brain. It has control over the complex process of receiving and transforming the information received from the retina of the eyes. The inner border of the two hemispheres is called the "limbic system," or "the thinking cap." It is a group of brain structures that have some influence over emotions and behavior. Two important parts of the system are the amygdala and the hippocampus. The first seems to control emotions; and the latter, memory.

The Complexity of the Brain

The brain is about the size of an average cantaloupe, or large grapefruit, and contains an estimated 100 billion nerve cells or neurons, which are the keys to the brain's communication system. If the nerve cells die or, for some reason, fail to function, the brain is in trouble. Each nerve cell has a long, tail-like extension called the "axon," which carries information from that cell to other cells by means of electrical impulses. Each axon may branch out into 10,000 terminals, and each terminal may reach out and connect with other cells. The body of each nerve cell is topped by a kind of tree-like extension, with numerous tiny branches called "dendrites," through which each nerve cell can receive messages from more than a thousand other cells. This is a mind-boggling and unbelievable intercommunication, which goes on every minute of our lives. As small as the brain is, it is estimated that it can store 100 trillion pieces of information.

It is in that incredibly complex organ that scientists are seeking the causes and cures for Alzheimer's and other dementias. Can man finally unravel the functions of that complex organ and discover the secrets of memory, intelligence, thinking, personality, behavior, and other human qualities? Can we not only discover the faults which produce dementia symptoms, but then devise a means of removing or subduing those faults and arrive at a cure?

I find some hope when I consider the astounding achievements in recent decades. If we can send men to the moon and back; if we can send a vehicle to the most remote planet and have it arrive on time, take pictures, and send them back; if we can unlock the secrets of the atom and use them to make bombs; if we can transplant a heart from one individual to another; and if we can operate on a fetus in the womb, I have hope that we will unravel the mysteries of the brain. This is the ultimate challenge of the mind of man.

The Brain as an Electrochemical Organ

To start the discussion of this aspect of the brain, I quote the following: "In Michelangelo's painting, 'The Creation of Adam,' the hands of God and Adam reach out to each other but do not touch as God gives Adam the divine spark creating the soul of man. Within the brain, a similar event occurs. Billions upon billions of nerve cells in the human brain make perhaps as many as a quadrillion connections. As each nerve cell reaches toward another, an earthly spark passes: an electrical and chemical impulse that enables us to think, feel, learn, remember, move, and sense the world around us. Flashing in intricate patterns from one neuron to the next, this electrochemical spark somehow builds awareness, giving man the power to contemplate his own existence. It is indeed a spark of life." [7]

In the brain, like the hand of God and the hand of Adam in the painting, the nerve cells do not actually touch each other, but messages pass from one cell to another as though they were on an electric wire. Between the cells, there is a tiny space called the "synaptic gap." Each cell generates electrical impulses and, when an impulse reaches the end of a cell, it triggers the release of chemical substances called neurotransmitters. These are discharged from the nerve endings into and across the synaptic gap to the receiving cell. In this manner, messages pass from one nerve cell to another. The neurotransmitters are, therefore, essential to the proper functioning of the brain. Faulty neurotransmission may be responsible for the loss of memory, the inability to think, and the unusual behavior of the victims of Alzheimer's.

Neuroscientists now know that there are many kinds of neurotransmitters, perhaps 200 or more, and different nerve cells in the network use different neurotransmitters. The neurotransmitter system which is believed to be concerned with memory and thought is called the "cholinergic system." This means that the cholinergic cells, which are concerned with memory and thinking, make use of the neurotransmitter acetylcholine in sending messages from one to the other. The transmission of a nerve impulse from one cell to another is an electrochemical

[7] Tolstar Books, *The Brain: Mystery Of Mind And Matter,* p. 37.

process. The axon, a long fiber extending from the body of the cell, conveys the impulse to neighboring cells. The transmission is done by means of a chemical chain reaction and, for the process to work properly, all links in the chain must be in place. It is in this unbelievably complex process, involving billions of cells, that scientists are looking for a possible cause and cure for Alzheimer's and related dementias.

How do we Know what we Know About the Brain?

Through the centuries, the brain has been a great mystery to philosophers, medical doctors, and mankind in general. Until recently, efforts to study the brain were handicapped by the inability to see the living brain in action. The traditional way of studying the brain was by autopsy upon death and, although much could be learned in that way, there was no way to see the living brain in action. Within the last quarter of a century, thanks to science and sophisticated technology, that has changed. In addition to the CAT scan, other sophisticated ways of viewing what is going on in the brain have been developed. One way is PET, Positron-Emission Tomography. It is a scanning technique that measures the body's uptake of radioactively labeled substances. PET provides a dynamic image of the brain's metabolic activity and has been useful in detecting Huntington's disease and Alzheimer's disease. PET has thus far been limited by its great costs, involving millions of dollars, and a number of skilled people, who are required to operate it. Another tool for studying the brain is NMR, Nuclear Magnetic Resonance. NMR gives an extremely clear picture of the biochemistry of the brain.

Through PET and NMR, it is possible to look through the skull and see the chemical and electrical activity of the living brain. Measuring these activities is a way of finding disorders and exploring the functions of the brain. These imaging methods, however, have not been able to contribute much to the diagnosis of Alzheimer's, although they can rule out other conditions that may cause Alzheimer-type symptoms.

Much excitement has come from the announcement of a new computer-enhanced X-ray technique, SPECT. SPECT is an acronym for Single Photon Emission Computed Tomography. Dr. Frederick J. Bonte, Director of the Nuclear Medicine Research Center at University of Texas Southwestern Medical Center in Dallas said, "SPECT may turn out to be the single most important imaging method we have to diagnose Alzheimer's." The procedure takes less than four minutes to perform and, at a cost of $450, it is relatively inexpensive.

Much research has been done during the last few years which has given rise to optimism among scientists. Time, and continued research, will, I hope eventually find a way to slow damage to nerve cells and to stop it altogether. ❧

```
┌─────────────────────┐
│      CHAPTER        │
│        ──           │
│        VI           │
│                     │
└─────────────────────┘
```

COPING WITH ALZHEIMER'S IN BESS
AND OLD AGE IN MYSELF

What Does Age Have to do With It?

My experience as a husband/caregiver for my wife with
Alzheimer's began in my late 70s, and lasted into the first year
of my 90s. My wife and I were both among the oldest of the old.
I do not know of another couple as old who has had a similar
tragedy. I have often wondered what, if anything, age has to do
with it. Does the caring for a spouse with Alzheimer's impose a
heavier physical, mental, and emotional burden on a person my
age than on a younger one? I know of no scientific evidence that
provides a definitive answer. Speaking from my personal experience and other scientific findings about the aging process, I am
convinced that age does have something to do with it. We do
know that the immune system weakens with age and that the
stress which falls on the caregiver may further weaken that system. Our overall fitness declines with age, and we have less
physical and emotional endurance. In my case, my wife and I
had been married for almost half a century, and to see her die a
lingering death was unbearable. Fortunately, there was no serious physical burden. Since I was in good health, I was able to
take over the household duties. My major problem was the ter-

rible mental and emotional stress that threatened my health and even my life. I had learned that it might take ten to 15 years, or even longer, for Alzheimer's to run its course. How could I, at the age of ninety, bear the terrible burden I was laboring under? In order to see that she got the best care possible, I must live as long as she was alive; I must preserve my own physical, mental, and emotional well-being. I then realized that I had to cope with two problems: how to withstand the mental and emotional burden of my wife's Alzheimer's and how to age successfully and live as long as possible. It was then that I began to seek whatever scientific evidence was available about the effects of age on the body and what, if anything, I could do to slow the aging process and preserve my good health.

Finding a Mechanism of Escape for my Mind

I began a search for a mental activity that would keep my mind off what was happening to Bess. The activity would have to be something profoundly interesting, meaningful, and mind-absorbing. I turned my thoughts to writing the story of my life and the struggle I had to get an education and make something of myself. One of my sisters had earlier suggested that I write down my life story for the family, but I had never found the time. I now had the time, and my present frustration reminded me of how I had overcome in my younger days what had then seemed impossible. The writing of *Where There's A Will There's A Way* was an enjoyable and inspiring experience, and helped me escape from the terrible frustration and tension under which I was living. It probably saved me from an emotional breakdown and from becoming a secondary victim of Alzheimer's.

There is no way a caregiver can rid his/her mind of all the mental and emotional stress which Alzheimer's imposes but, in my case, writing eased the stress somewhat and made it bearable. I would not suggest that all caregivers undertake to write a book as a coping technique. Some may lack the interest, the time, or the ability. I do suggest, however, that the caregiver find an interesting, meaningful, mental activity to keep the brain busy and functioning at its optimum level. That will be helpful in coping with both Alzheimer's and old age. So much the better if the activity is challenging. Everyone must keep a positive attitude, as well as an open and flexible mind in dealing with either or both of those problems. Writing a book just happened to be my way.

Having written the story of my early life and my struggle to get an education, I turned to writing the story of my professional life, titled *Forty Years in the Classroom*. The writing of that book was also an interesting experience and was equally helpful in bearing my burden. After I completed the story of my entire life, Bess was worse, and the long-lasting burden on me was becoming evident. What should I do next? By that time, I had read all I could find on Alzheimer's and old age. Why not write the story of my experience with Alzheimer's disease, how it had affected both Bess and me, and how I had coped with it thus far? My experience and coping methods might be helpful and encouraging to other caregivers.

My writing was done amidst many interruptions. Since Bess could no longer read nor watch TV, she simply sat and watched me as I typed. I could not get away from her into another room. Just to see her sitting and staring at me was difficult to bear. Frequently, she would say, "Let's do something," or "Let's go somewhere," or "Let's get dinner." I would then stop writing, and we would play an old game, *Aggravation*, which she had not completely forgotten. Sometimes, we would go for a ride. She could not walk very far without complaining of her feet. She would often say, "Let's go see Mamie," her sister, who lived 15 miles away. We might have already been there that day, but she would have forgotten. Occasionally, she would pick up a page which I had written and ask, "Why are you writing this? Nobody is going to read it." When I started writing about Alzheimer's, I did not use our names. We were "Jack and Jill."

Finding Ways to Cope with Old Age and Preserve My Good Health

Keeping the brain active and functioning well is extremely important for the Alzheimer's caregiver. Physical and mental exercise is essential if the brain is to remain sharp and functioning well in old age. The other vital organs—the heart, the lungs, the immune system, the muscles, and the joints—are also essential to good health and a long life. Physical exercise and a proper diet play important roles in keeping all these organs and systems functioning properly.

Dr. Robert N. Butler said, "If exercise could be packaged in a pill, it could be the most widely prescribed medicine on the market." Some form of regular exercise is essential to maintain good health and to withstand the strains and tensions which fall on the caregiver. Before Bess went to live in the nursing home, I could find neither the time or the opportunity to exercise regularly. I was able, in season, to garden, and do the yard work. I bought a stationary bike and put it in the basement, but when I went down to use it, Bess would come and ask me to be with her, saying she was lonely. It was only after she went to the nursing home that I was able to adopt a regular program of walking three miles at a rapid pace of 100 to 120 steps per minute, three to five times per week. Although I had been able to do in-house exercise, it was not until Bess was in the nursing home that I was able to work out a comprehensive and regular series of exercises, performed in the bed and on the floor.

Several times each week, I worked through my exercise program to strengthen every joint and muscle in my body, from my toes to my fingers, with special emphasis on the lower back and stomach muscles. I had, for a number of years, been troubled with lower-back pain, from which I am now free. Except for the purchase of the stationary bike and two five-pound weights, my exercise program has cost me nothing except the time spent, but it has been invaluable. I have completely rid myself of the lower-back pain, improved my heart, lungs, muscles, and joints; I sleep better and feel better. My weight is within five pounds of what it was when Bess and I were married in 1927. My strong heart has kept my brain supplied with the necessary oxygen to keep it functioning well. Regular exercise has helped me to bear the strains and tensions under which I lived. It has helped me to grow old very successfully and to preserve my physical, mental, and emotional well-being. Without the writing and a regular exercise program, it is doubtful that I could have lived through the long years during which Bess had Alzheimer's.

Caregiving for an Alzheimer's patient has been called a 36-hour day. To cope successfully, the caregiver needs help from outside the family. Daycare centers and support groups are the best sources of help. I was a caregiver for Bess for about eight years before there was any such help available in my community.

I finally discovered ACTO (Alzheimer's Caregivers Time Out), a volunteer daycare center, which offered care once each week for four hours. This provided a few hours of valuable time out for me, and was the best help for Bess I was able to find. It served both of us well until I placed her in the nursing home. Up to that point, however, it was impossible for me to attend a support group regularly. Afterward, I **was** able to attend a support group, where I found the friendship, the understanding of other caregivers, and the moral support I badly needed.

In most cases where a husband and wife live in a home or apartment without the presence of another family member, a sense of social isolation becomes an ever-present and serious problem for the caregiver. It is perhaps worse for the husband than for the wife. My experience has led me to believe that the older the caregiver, the worse the problem. One of the hardest problems of growing old is the loss of lifelong friends. During Bess' long illness, I lost all except one of my best longtime friends and professional colleagues. Those losses came one by one, over a 15-year period. Because of age and Bess' illness, it was difficult to make new friends. Fortunately, I live in a wonderful neighborhood, where I am surrounded by good, friendly neighbors. I have many good friends among the members of the support group. Frequently, I have lunch with a former, but much younger colleague, who was also a professor of political science. I also have occasional lunches with the widow of a longtime friend. Since she was an English teacher, she edits my writing. I meet frequently with other friends for short talks. These social and intellectual relationships are invaluable, and keep me from feeling isolated. Such relationships are great sources of inspiration, learning, and the positive outlook which make life worth living. Don't overlook the fact that, if you are to **have** good neighbors, you must also **be** a good neighbor and good friend. Don't allow yourself to become a recluse and lose one of the great values and joys of life.

Humor has played an important role in my efforts to cope with Alzheimer's and in my efforts to come to terms with old age. Bess had a great sense of humor and found a lot of fun in life. One of the reasons I loved and married her was her sense of humor. It was one of the human qualities which even Alzheimer's did not destroy. She still had that sense of humor until shortly before she died. One of the great and most effective coping weapons for caregivers is humor. It is often difficult to find, but I was sometimes able to do it. The reader will find many examples of humor throughout this book, and Bess herself was the source of much of it.

Finally, a young-at-heart feeling and a positive attitude served me well as coping devices. Such feelings and attitudes are difficult for an old person to maintain; yet it can be done. Reliving my life from memory and writing about it gave me a sense of satisfaction with my past. Cooking, gardening, and exercise also gave me a great sense of pleasure and accomplishment and kept me feeling young-at-heart. ↔

CHAPTER
VII

THE ROLE OF HOUSEHUSBAND

When Bess lost the ability to perform her duties as a house-wife, I became a househusband, doing what she, as the house-wife, had always done. For most men that would be a drastic change in their lifestyle and, for many, it would be impossible. Fortunately, I did not come to my new role without experience and interest. My main difficulty came from Bess, who was so obsessed with cooking that she could not give it up and permit me do it. Her interference with my efforts to cook became the most frustrating part of my role as househusband.

My interest and experience in cooking go back to my two years in junior college, where I worked to pay my expenses. Cooking, baking, washing dishes, and janitorial services were all performed by students who worked their way through college. During my first year I was assigned to the breakfast crew, who prepared breakfast every morning for a large student body. Among the items served were old-fashioned white biscuits which I prepared and baked in two large woodburning ovens. Having done that every morning for nine months, I became an all-around biscuit-maker and could, with some justification, claim to have made more biscuits than any woman in the entire South. After Bess and I were married, I never had the opportunity to put that particular expertise to use; not since my college days have I made and baked an old-fashioned white biscuit.

Frustrations as a Cook and Caregiver

Observing an excellent cook for 50 years taught me a lot about the art of cooking. My past experience and the knowledge I had gained from Bess served me well when I was forced to assume the role of househusband.

In coming to terms with old age and coping with dementia in Bess, it was essential that I find meaning and, if possible, a sense of achievement in everything I did. Cooking became an excellent coping technique for me. I ceased buying Christmas gifts for family members and friends. Instead, I baked a variety of fruit and nut breads, rum cakes, wine cakes, and cookies, and made jams and jellies, all of which they enjoyed more than any article I could afford to buy. I have never yet had a gift brought back after Christmas for exchange! To avoid the rush just before Christmas and to help me through a period of depression, I often baked and froze breads and cakes at various times during the year. On many occasions, I have done these things in the middle of the night when it was impossible to sleep.

The most frustrating daily activity I had as Bess' caregiver was having to cook. Every day, and every meal except breakfast, I went through the frustrating process of preparing our meals. She could not give up the idea that she should cook, nor could she accept the fact that I was a competent cook; yet she never refused to eat what I cooked.

Bess was not only an excellent cook, but she had mastered the art of cooking without burning food. She did, however, have on the wall of the breakfast room a little plaque which read: "It is better to have cooked and burned than never to have cooked at all." When scorched food began to appear on our table almost every day, it was a definite sign that something was wrong. Although I made no complaint, and she offered no excuses, the burned food continued to appear. Finally, one day she called me in from the yard to see that she had burned the bottom out of the kettle while boiling water, and the molten metal had scarred the stovetop. I knew then that it was time for me to help her with the cooking, or even to take the full responsibility for it.

I felt like the young man in the maternity ward at the hospital, waiting for his wife to deliver their first baby. They had been married about a year, and the young wife had not yet mastered the art of cooking without burning. Two older men were also there, awaiting the birth of a baby. The nurse, who thought she might have some fun, took a little black baby and asked one of the older men, "Is this yours?" He replied, "No, ma'ame." She took it to the other man, and he said, "No ma'ame, that's not mine." She then took it to the young man and asked, "Is this yours?" He took a look and said, "Could be. She's burned everything else."

When the doctor learned that I had become the cook in my family, he said to me, "You must help your wife lose some weight. She is much too heavy." I promised to do my best. Bess had been overweight all her life and had tried a number of times to lose weight. Although she had been successful on a few occasions, she had never been able to keep the weight down for more than a short while. Along with the dementia symptoms, her weight began to increase.

Since I knew that achieving my goal would require time, I was not interested in any of the highly advertised quick-fix programs. I, therefore, turned to the recommendations of the American Heart Association and the Institute for Cancer Research for help in designing a diet to reduce her weight and preserve her health. In addition to those requirements, the diet had to be appetizing to both of us. I reduced our consumption of beef, pork, and eggs and increased our consumption of chicken, fish, and turkey, which we both enjoyed. I omitted salt, reduced fat and sugar, and discontinued fried foods. I baked or broiled our meats and, where possible, steamed our vegetables, or served them raw. I increased our consumption of vegetables and served fruit or juice three times a day. For desserts, I reduced the sugar content, and served skimmed milk.

Bess could not understand why I cut the fat from meat and denied her salt. She would often salt her meat or vegetables three or four times during a meal. It required time but, after 18 months, I had achieved my goal. Bess had lost forty pounds, and I had lost fifteen. If I left Bess alone in the house, regardless of the time of day, she would immediately go to the kitchen and start cooking. I came in from the yard once and found her frying two chicken breasts which I planned to bake for dinner. The electric unit was on high, the chicken was already burned black, and the grease was popping all over the stovetop. Thereafter, I never left her alone again without first cutting the power to the stove and oven; but that did not solve the problem. A few days later, she called me in from the yard and said, "Come and show me how to start a fire to cook this fish." I had bought two salmon steaks for dinner that evening and Bess, thinking they were too thick to cook, had cut them into shreds. When she turned the stove on and it failed to get hot, she could only think of starting a fire. I blew up. "Oh my God, Bess! Why in hell don't you get out of the kitchen and leave the cooking to me?" Following that incident, I not only cut off the power, but I took all the meat to an extra refrigerator in the basement. She would then call me from the yard or garden to say, "We must go to the grocery store to get something for dinner."

When I prepared meals, she was in the kitchen every minute, telling me how to do it. If I was preparing chicken to bake, for example, she would complain when I trimmed the fat off. "You can't cook it without the fat. It won't be fit to eat." If I were cooking canned green beans, she would insist that I put a piece of fat pork with them for seasoning. That was what she did when we were first married, but she had long ago substituted vegetable oil for pork.

Since we were fond of corn muffins, I often baked them to eat with fish. I used ready-mixed meal, but she could never understand why I did not put soda and salt in the mix. She would ask, "Have you put the soda in? Have you turned the oven on? Have you greased the muffin pans?"

I tried to give her something to do to keep her out of the kitchen. If I asked her to set the table, she did not know where to find the dishes or the silver. She would often ask, "Is Daddy going to eat with us?" or "Is Mama going to eat with us?" Whenever I asked her to take the dishes out of the dishwasher, she did not know where to put them. If I asked her to peel a potato, she might start, but could not finish it. When asked to pour the tea or the milk, she might pour the milk into the tea glasses and the tea into the milk glasses. She would often look in the oven to see what was cooking, then she would change the temperature setting, or take the food from the oven.

There were no problems at breakfast. I arose early and had breakfast ready by the time she came to the breakfast room but, for lunch and dinner, I lived through frustration, anger, and sorrow for her. If she had just sat down and let me alone, I would have enjoyed cooking. I knew that she could not help doing what she was doing, but that did not prevent my frustration and anger. She would not leave the kitchen if I asked her to. I would often get behind her and push her out to the breakfast room, but that did not stop her tongue. As much as I loved Bess, and as happy as our married life had been, it was becoming difficult to live with her.

Bess had driven a car for more than 40 years and, for a number of years, had had her own car. She had a perfect driving record, no speeding tickets, no parking tickets, not even a dent in a fender of her car. Driving her car was a much-cherished privilege. After I retired, we agreed to sell her car and use one car instead of two. We continued our practice of taking turns at the wheel on long trips. We had known many cases where the husband, after retirement, did all the driving and, through lack of use, the wife lost her ability to drive. When the husband died, she was left handicapped and unable to drive until she learned again. Bess had asked me not to do that to her, and I had promised that I would not. The time came, however, when she could no longer drive without endangering herself, or others, and I had to break my promise. There was no way to explain that it was for her safety as well as mine. She thought me a male chauvinist who was denying her the cherished right to drive. **That,** she thought, was contrary to the behavior of Bill, the husband she had lived with for so long. Being a strong-willed and determined person, she assumed a role which I could not deny her, that of a "backseat driver," a role she did not give up, even after I placed her in a nursing home. If I took her out for a ride and she saw me driving 40-miles-an-hour in a 35-mile zone, she would remind me. If I stopped at a red light in a left lane to make a turn, she would often say, "You had better turn on your signal." Of course, it was already flashing, but from the passenger seat, she had not noticed. Such an expression of mental acuity on her part was simply unbelievable. How could one who had lost her memory, her ability to think, and other mental abilities manage to perceive the situation and express a warning? She often paid no attention to a red light; she forgot how to change gears; she did not remember to turn on the windshield wipers if it started raining, and she did not know how to turn on the lights as darkness approached. If she drove alone, she got lost. If she went to the grocery store with me, which was just three-quarters of a mile away, she did not know the direction home and would say to me, "This is not the way home." She would make a left turn in the face of oncoming traffic and scare the life out of me. In the interest of safety, I had no choice — I had to break my promise. Following one dangerous incident, I said to her, "Bess, do you know what might have happened?" She replied, "I don't care what might have happened." That did it! I never allowed her to have the car keys again.

Bess also had her fantasies. We had bought a cemetery lot 15 years earlier. I thought the matter was settled but one day she said to me, "Let's sell our cemetery lot and buy one in the cemetery over on the mountain." There is no mountain near Atlanta, except Stone Mountain, and there is no cemetery there. When I asked her why she did not want to be buried in the lot we already had, she told me that trees had grown up around it. I replied, "Well, let's go see." There were trees scattered through the cemetery, but none near our lot. When we saw what a beautiful place it was, she seemed satisfied, and we returned home. A few days later, she again raised the subject and insisted that we buy a new lot over on the mountain. Finally, I decided to sell our original lot and buy one in another cemetery, where our daughter and her husband have a lot. That seemed to please Bess.

A month later, she brought up the subject again, and told me that our lot had been moved into what she called a "wet, swampy area." I could not convince her that the lot could not have been changed without our consent, nor could I get the subject off her mind. Again, I took her to see it and she seemed satisfied. Less than ten days later, however, she raised the same doubts again. Once again, I took her to see it and again, she appeared satisfied, and we returned home. A few days later, she again insisted that we move our lot and I told her firmly that this was out of the question. She seemed disappointed but, after a few weeks, she forgot the matter and did not bring it up again. The controversy over the cemetery lot illustrates the point that victims of dementia are not rational. It is impossible to reason with them. There is no way to explain that they are wrong or mistaken, or that what they believe to be true cannot be so. They have lost their rationality and can no longer use reason to understand a situation.

Bess had also lost her social abilities and felt ill at ease and insecure in the presence of other people, even friends and relatives. When we drove 250 miles to North Carolina to visit relatives and friends, she became unhappy within a short while and wanted to return home. If asked why, she would say, "I must cook dinner," or, "We did not bring sleeping garments to spend the night." If we went to a family gathering or a Christmas party at the home of our daughter, she became unhappy and wanted to go home. Soon, we were cut off from all social contacts. She felt secure only at home with me but, even there, she was unhappy and would ask me to take her to see her sister Mamie. When I took her to see Mamie, the two would not speak more than half a dozen words to each other. A short while after we had returned home, she would ask again to go to see Mamie. When I told her we had already been there, she would not believe it, and would call me a liar.

Bess lost her knowledge of the relationship of Estelle and her husband, John. Because I was in the hospital for a few days, she stayed with them. When Estelle showed her mother the bedroom where she would sleep, Bess asked, "Where are you and John going to sleep?" Estelle told her they would sleep in the master bedroom. To this simple statement, Bess replied, with deep concern, "You mean you are going to sleep together?"

Estelle said, "Yes." Then Bess said, "Not at my house do you sleep together!" Estelle explained to her that she and John had been married for 30 years and said to her, "You and Daddy sleep together." That did not satisfy her, though and she insisted that Estelle sleep with her.

On a visit to see me at the hospital, Estelle pushed the elevator button for the fifth floor, to go to my room. When they reached the third floor, a man entered and pushed the button for the sixth floor. Bess did not understand and said to him, "Don't do that." Somewhat startled, he pushed the same button again. She said, "I told you not to do that. You will break this thing, and we will get stuck and never get down."

Reaching My Limits as a Caregiver

As Bess lost her memory, her self-initiative, and her independence, she turned more and more to me and home for security and a feeling of safety. Away from home, among other people, she felt insecure and afraid. At home she felt lonely without my presence. I could not get away from her for a minute, even to take a walk, to mow the grass, to work in the garden, to work in my shop in the basement, not even go to another room in the house. If I went to the basement, she would come down and say, "I am lonely. Come upstairs and be with me." If I went to the yard and began mowing the grass, she would come and ask, "When are we going to cook dinner? What are we going to eat? There is nothing in the refrigerator." I would assure her that we would find something and that I would quit mowing at the proper time to prepare it. Within ten or 15 minutes, she would be back asking the same question. In the evening, she wanted to go to bed early, about eight-thirty or nine o'clock, but would not go without me. The only way I could find time to read or write was to go to bed with her, stay until she was asleep, and then quietly

63

slip out. If she should awaken, she would be after me and demand that I come to bed. She could not, or would not, take a nap in the afternoon, nor would she permit me to do so. If I should fall asleep in my chair after dinner, she would arouse me. I became for her a kind of "security blanket."

Her feelings toward me, however, were ambivalent, a mixed, love-hate feeling. Despite her love for me and her dependence on me for companionship to escape her loneliness, she would accuse me of lying to her, of mistreating her, of doing for myself what I wanted to do, but refusing to do what she wanted me to do. That both hurt and angered me, although I knew that she was not responsible for what she was saying. Her former strong will had become stubbornness, and her former outspokenness had become denunciations and accusations. She had lost her self-control.

She became uncooperative and obstinate. Once, after I had made a doctor's appointment for her, I had to cancel it because she absolutely refused to go. In my effort to reduce her weight, I needed to check it frequently, but she would refuse to get on the bathroom scale. Once, as she stood next to the toilet, I managed to get both of her feet on the scale, and the reading indicated she had lost 50 pounds. When I looked up, she had both hands on the toilet, lifting her weight off the scales. That was evidence of a surviving bit of knowledge and understanding somewhere in her brain.

Instances of extreme stubbornness and denunciation were many, but I will relate one which I shall never forget. She had become urinary incontinent and had to wear Depends pads. She never failed to wash her face before going to bed. She did not need a shower every day, but she did need to wash more than her face. If I asked her to wash under her arms and between her legs, she would say, "You get in there and wash under your own arms and between your own legs ... "

Although I used all of my persuasive powers to get her to take a shower, she was equally as stubborn about it. I would turn on the water and adjust the temperature, offer to get into the shower with her, to wash her back, or to help her take a tub bath. Often, nothing I tried would work, and she would go for days without taking any kind of bath. One Saturday night as we prepared for bed, I said, "This is Saturday night. Suppose we take a shower?" She was sitting on the side of the bed, entirely unclothed, ready to step into the shower stall. She said, "I don't need a bath. I had one last night." It had been ten days or longer since she had been in the shower. I said, "Oh, come on. We will feel better and sleep better. Do you want to go first, or shall I?" She said, "I don't need a bath, I am just flat not going to take a bath, and you can't make me." She continued, "I am damned tired of your telling me to do what I don't want to do. You treat me like I am a dog. You have always done that." That was the most violent outburst of anger, defiance, and accusation I had ever heard from her. It surprised and angered me. I did not want to strike her, hurt her, or abuse her in any way, but I walked over to her, took her by the hair of the head and said, "Honey, you are going to have a shower tonight." I led her to the shower. There was vigorous objection, but it was entirely vocal. "Damn you, Bill. Turn me loose." Once in the shower stall, she stood back as far from the shower as possible, with the water striking only her lower legs and feet. I closed the shower door and walked out. A few minutes later, I looked in, and she was standing under the shower, apparently enjoying it. Soon, I heard her turn off the water, open the shower door, and say, "Bill, come dry my back." She had entirely forgotten the means I had used to get her into the shower.

I was surprised and angry with myself for what I had done. How could I do such a thing to Bess? I have cried, laughed, and cursed a number of times over that experience. Had a cartoonist seen it, he might have drawn a picture with the caption, "Retired college professor uses caveman method to give his wife a shower."

I hesitated and debated with myself about making this incident public. I have since learned that I am not the only man who has tried force to get his wife to take a shower. A woman I know went one night to sit with the wife of a minister, who had to be away on business. The wife had Alzheimer's, and the woman asked him about bruises she saw on the patient's arms. He confessed that they were the result of his efforts to get his wife to the bathroom to take a shower. It is a striking illustration of what a dementing disease can do to its victim and the caregiver, even a loving husband to a loving wife.

I had carried the combined load of househusband and full-time caregiver for about eight years, and those had been years of mixed feelings—love, compassion, frustration, grief, anger, helplessness, and tension. How long can a man in his 80's hold up under that kind of burden? I had driven a car for more than 66 years without a ticket for speeding, but I finally got one. During those 66 years, I had never had an accident for which I was judged in the wrong. I finally had one. I could no longer go to sleep at night before using an electric vibrator to relieve my tense stomach muscles. The dementia which was destroying Bess was also destroying me. For both her sake and mine, I had to find some way to save myself. Finally, my determination never to put her in a nursing home was broken, and I realized that it was only a matter of time. It was then that I began to look for some way to delay that decision as long as possible.

I took Bess to two different daycare centers, both of which were just getting started. Neither was satisfactory, nor would Bess stay. I then learned of ACTO (an acronym for Alzheimer's

Caregiver's Time Out). The name conveyed what I was looking for—time out. If my time out was to be worthwhile to me, I had to know that it would be meaningful to Bess also. We both needed time away from each other. If ACTO could meet our needs, it was a wonderful discovery, and I had found a temporary solution to my problem. ⟂

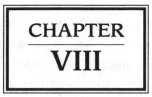

CHAPTER
VIII

ACTO – ALZHEIMER'S CAREGIVERS TIMEOUT DAYCARE CENTER

Our conventional nursing homes were designed to care for patients whose primary needs were for basic skilled nursing and medical care. However, with the increase of Alzheimer's Disease among our aging population, a new type of patient is entering our nursing homes, whose needs are far more demanding. For the most part, conventional nursing homes lack the facilities, the equipment, and the staff needed to deal effectively with the needs of Alzheimer's patients. The majority of patients are cared for at home, by a member of the family (often an elderly spouse, who is ill-prepared to serve their needs). Moreover, the effects on the family caregiver are often so emotionally and physically devastating that he or she needs moral support and help from outside the family to avoid becoming a secondary victim. Despite their loss of such human qualities as memory, the ability to think, self-initiative, and self-reliance, the victims of this disease still have human needs which must be met and served. They also retain certain abilities, which, with the help of knowledgeable people, can help relieve them of boredom, confusion, fear, and social isolation.

There is hope that a cure will be found for Alzheimer's disease at some time in the future but, in the meantime, we must devise better and more humane methods of caring for its victims. In response to the growing awareness of the effects of Alzheimer's, there are a number of new efforts underway. Among them are daycare centers designed to meet their special needs, in-home respite services, personal care homes, separate Alzheimer's units in nursing homes, and family support groups to serve the needs of the family caregiver. This chapter is devoted to a discussion and evaluation of a volunteer daycare center where Bess found better care for her needs than at any other place.

ACTO: Alzheimer's Caregivers Time-Out

ACTO is sponsored by the North DeKalb County Lioness Club near Atlanta, Georgia. The Center provides a recreation and socialization program in a safe non-threatening environment for persons with a diagnosis of dementia. The primary purpose is to give caregivers a few hours respite from their "36-Hour Day," as described by Nancy L. Mace and Peter V. Rabins in their book, *The 36-Hour Day.*

The volunteers are all highly dedicated people, who have had no professional training for a caregiving role. Through reading, observation, and firsthand experience, they have become aware of the cruel and devastating impact Alzheimer's disease has on the victim and caregiver. Being compassionate and caring people, a group of Lions and Lionesses traveled at their own expense to Kentucky where an ACTO center was already in operation. After several weeks of observation and study, they returned to establish such a center here.

Some Special Features of ACTO

ACTO is designed to provide recreational activities and meaningful social relationships for participants. Perhaps the single most important feature is the one-to-one ratio of caregiver to participant. I have been there when there were more volunteers

70

than participants. The one-to-one ratio helps the volunteer to learn more about the individual and makes it possible for each participant to receive individual attention. Without the dedication and presence of a number of volunteers and the financial support of the Lioness Club, it would be too costly to maintain such a ratio.

Another significant and important feature of ACTO is the presence of male volunteers. It is possible, of course, to conduct an effective daycare program without the aid of men, but they do add to the social value of the ACTO program. Male victims of dementia who are brought to ACTO may feel more comfortable in a group with men volunteers. Some men need assistance in going to the toilet, and feel more comfortable being helped by male volunteers. They may respond to certain games and activities more readily with the encouragement of men. On one occasion, the leader of a daycare program found an amusing role for the men. The women volunteers brought out-of-date women's clothing—dresses, hats, and shoes. A 'fashion show' with a difference was staged— the men were dressed in women's clothing and they paraded in front of the group. A vote was taken and a winner proclaimed, to the amusement of all.

A third important feature of ACTO is that each daily program is planned and administered by a single leader, who is not responsible for more than one program per month. This arrangement distributes the burden and allows sufficient time for the preparation of the program. It also creates variety and a better quality of programs. Preparing and conducting a successful program requires knowledge, imagination, ingenuity, skill, and hard work. I remained and participated in a few programs, just to observe firsthand their nature and quality and Bess' response. Knowing that she was in the hands of people who could engage her meaningfully made my time out even more valuable.

71

Meeting the Social Needs of the Participants

Most victims of Alzheimer's have a sense of social isolation. They develop a feeling of insecurity, loneliness, and fear. They need the human touch and human relationships. Having been a very sociable person, Bess was left insecure and fearful in the presence of others after she lost her social skills, such as the ability to remember names, to take the initiative, and to contribute to the conversation. ACTO met her needs in this respect exceptionally well. When she arrived for a meeting, she was always greeted by volunteers with hugs, kisses, handshakes, and expressions of endearment. She got a tender, loving, human touch from friendly people. She did not say a word, but her smile and the expression on her face were proof of her feelings. She could not remember the name of a single person, nor could she remember having been there the week before, but she loved it and got the emotional lift which she needed. She did not react as the former Bess would have done; she did not reach out to other people, nor did she say, "I am happy to see you." Her smile was her only response. She lost, for a time, her sense of aloneness and insecurity, her sense of being socially isolated, and gained a sense of belonging with a group of friendly people. Her psychosocial relief, with few exceptions, lasted through the program, until she saw me arrive to take her home. She then wanted to go home without delay.

Following her welcoming, she was led to a table where there were snacks, such as popcorn, potato chips, and cheese puff balls. Seated at the table with other participants, the volunteers gently stimulated conversation. Contrary to her former self, she seldom, if ever, volunteered any statements of her own, but would answer questions if asked.

Everyone brought a sandwich for lunch, and ACTO provided tea or coffee and a dessert. The lunch hour was a social occasion and again volunteers helped patients engage in light conversation. Throughout the program, Bess was in close touch with one or more volunteers and was given encouragement and praise in her activities.

Meeting the Recreational Needs of the Participants

ACTO meets in the activities building of a local church. There is nothing homelike about it, but it is comfortable during both summer and winter and is large enough for activities. It has a kitchen, a piano, restrooms for both men and women, and enough tables and chairs for any program. It is adequate for the once-a-week four-hour session.

Their programs consist of activities which help to stimulate and utilize the participants' remaining capacities. The aim is to give them something meaningful to do within their abilities. Throughout the day, most victims of Alzheimer's need, and want, something to do to relieve their boredom and frustration, but they need to be directed and guided. Since their abilities and interests vary, preparing programs to meet their needs is a challenge. Among the recreational activities are: a short period of simple and easy-to-do physical exercise, a sing-a-long, volleyball, pitching a bean bag, horseshoes, pitching a basketball through a hoop, bingo, a game called "Finish-the-Proverb," spelling matches, simple crafts, making decorations for Easter, Valentine's Day, Thanksgiving, and Christmas, and making scrapbooks. Once or twice each year, there is a fashion show or a game of Pin-the-Tail-on-the-Donkey. Many games were made competitive between either individuals or groups, and small prizes were given to the winners. The program moved rapidly, so that there were few idle moments during the four-hour session.

I was once shown some scrapbooks, one made by Bess and one by another woman. Each was given a loose-leaf notebook, with a title written on the front, and chapter headings written inside. They were given a number of old magazines, a pair of scissors, and a tube of paste, and were instructed to clip from the magazine pictures to represent the chapter headings. Each had to use his or her mind to find and choose the pictures most representative of the titles and cut-and-paste the pictures on the appropriate pages. The title of the book given to Bess was "My Life". The chapter headings were: "My Childhood," "My Father and Mother," "My School Days," "My First Sweetheart," "My Husband," "His Family," "My Favorite Foods," "Our Home," "Our Car," and "My Next Husband." Bess made a very good selection of pictures and did a perfect job of clipping and pasting. I was a little puzzled about her next husband, for she had selected the pictures of two very handsome men. I liked her selection better, however, than what I saw in another woman's book. For her next husband, she had selected the picture of a big tom cat wearing a black bow tie.

Music and obviously humor, are not overlooked. Since there is a piano in the building and a pianist among the volunteers, there is always a musical element in the program. They sing a number of old, familiar songs, which everyone seems to enjoy. Once, for Bess and me, they sang "My Wild Irish Rose," a favorite song during our courting days. It was not unusual to see volunteers and participants dancing together during the musical part of the program.

From the beginning to the end of the program, humor and laughter abound. At the beginning, the leader may call on everyone to relate the most amusing thing he or she has seen or experienced since the last meeting. This opens the way for humorous incidents or jokes to begin the program. Some special features may be planned with humor as the main objective, like the fashion show mentioned earlier. I have been surprised by how well Bess and many other victims of dementia have retained a sense of humor, in spite of the loss of memory and other cognitive abilities.

The Limits and Possibilities of the Volunteer Approach

The volunteers at ACTO had an excellent program, a place where Bess could find a few hours of meaningful social activities once each week. Their objectives were sound—to sustain an optimal quality of life for patients for a few hours each week, and to provide relief for family caregivers. Their programs were based on concepts that the victims of Alzheimer's need, most of all, something worthwhile to do during the day, and social interaction with friendly people, to enable them to retain some sense of self-worth and security. ACTO was the only place I found that could provide for Bess, and others like her, what they really needed.

The time out which ACTO made possible was also valuable to me. It allowed me a few much-needed hours away from Bess. I could go to the barber shop without fear of leaving her alone. If my time out were to be really helpful, I needed to know that she was in the care of well-informed, dedicated, and friendly people who could help her find a few hours of the kind of life she needed. If they had been able to do this five days a week, I could have delayed the nursing home decision for months or, perhaps, years.

The real difficulty is in finding enough qualified and dedicated people who can, or will, spend the time to engage in such a program. This kind of intensive program is a burnout activity, which demands so much of the leader that she cannot conduct the program every day. Once a week is invaluable to the caregiver and the person with Alzheimer's disease, but it is not enough. How can we find enough volunteers to carry the heavy load, maintain the high ratio of volunteer-to-participant, and keep the program operating more days per week? It puts an extremely valuable service within reach of many who cannot afford the charges of the average daycare center.

Despite its limitations, I can recommend ACTO, without reservation, to other civic clubs and churches as a possible way to render a much-needed service to the increasing number of families who are caught in the devastating impact of a cruel dementia. With a growing awareness of the nature and gravity of the problem, perhaps we will find enough caring, empathetic, and dedicated people who will follow the example of ACTO as a kind of mission to improve the quality of life for a growing number of our elderly.

Objectives and Methods of a Humane Program of Caring

The primary objective of an Alzheimer's patient-care program should be to help its victims have meaningful and enjoyable lives for as long as possible, within the limits of their surviving mental and physical abilities. Achieving this objective requires caregivers who understand their needs and their surviving abilities, and who are able to devise and implement a recreational and social program to meet those needs. The basic-care nurses, while skilled, have neither the training nor the time to do this. We need a corps of caregivers, trained specifically to meet the needs of Alzheimer's victims to do it effectively.

Jitka M. Zgola, author of the valuable little guide book *Doing Things*, describes the concepts and philosophy of a successful daycare center as follows:

"We all have an inherent need to do things. We do things to define ourselves as individuals, to exert control over our environment, and to develop and secure meaningful relationships with others. Alzheimer's disease gradually erodes a person's ability to engage in many of the activities that fulfill these psychosocial needs."

The "Day Away" daycare center in Ottawa, Canada, is a good example of the kind of program required if we are to effectively meet the recreational and social needs of Alzheimer's patients. The "Day Away" program is in session throughout the entire day, four days per week, and serves a total of 32 people, eight per day. It uses both paid and volunteer staff, two staff members and four volunteers for each group of eight clients. Although the ratios may vary depending on the type of activity and the needs of the clients, it should always be sufficient to provide the initiative, leadership, and social stimulation which the clients need.

The "Day Away" programs consist of a variety of physical and social activities. The patients play games, exercise, prepare and serve the noon meal, hold sing-a-longs, engage in hobbies, take walks and have special programs for birthdays and holidays. There are also woodworking projects just for men.

The primary purpose is to keep the patients busy at activities throughout the day and to maintain meaningful social relationships. The result is an enjoyable day in the lives of the patients, which relieves them of their idleness and sense of social isolation. ❧

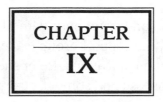

CHAPTER IX

ALZHEIMER SUPPORT GROUPS

The effects of Alzheimer's disease on its victims are so cruel and devastating that it has created caring problems different in some respects from those caused by other deadly diseases. The effects on the victims are more difficult for caregivers to cope with emotionally and physically. Caring for its victims is often long-term and financially burdensome. It is a new and unfamiliar kind of care which we are unable to handle effectively. Perhaps seventy percent of Alzheimer's patients are cared for at home, many of them by an elderly wife, husband or daughter. The burden on the caregiver is often so exhausting that, without help, the caregiver often becomes a secondary victim of the disease. It was out of this realization that the idea of a community organization composed of family caregivers developed into the Alzheimer's support group as the most logical instrument for helping caregivers. It is based on the principle of self-help and the belief that those who have firsthand knowledge of the disease and its effects are best qualified to provide the kind of help required by family caregivers.

The Importance of Leadership

During the last five years I have attended five different support groups. All have been very successful. Their success has been due in large part to their leaders.

In addition to firsthand experience with Alzheimer's as a caregiver or as a nurse, the support group leader must possess certain other important qualifications. He or she should have broad knowledge of the disease and some acquaintance with the literature, as well as awareness of ongoing research and experimentation. There are also certain personal qualities which are important. The leader should be a friendly, empathetic, and an outgoing person who can relate to caregivers. He or she should be able to make members feel at ease and comfortable with each other so that they will talk freely about their problems. This is essential if the support group is to function well. The leader should know how to conduct and guide a group discussion in order to stimulate participation by each member. It is important that the leader create an atmosphere in which each member feels secure and comfortable in expressing his or her feelings and experiences.

The Round Table Discussion Procedure

As members of the group arrive, they find and pin on name tags, engage in conversation, and partake of refreshments such as coffee, cookies, or cake. Books and literature from the Alzheimer's Association are usually available. This information helps keep caregivers current on all matters related to the disease.

In these groups, the round table discussion procedure is the most usual and the most helpful part of the program. Several times a year, however, we had an outside speaker from the medical profession, the legal profession or other area of interest. For example, we had a pathologist talk about autopsy, its importance, and the procedure involved. An attorney spoke about living wills, the durable power of attorney, and other legal matters of concern to caregivers. A pathologist, a social worker, and a recreation director also came to our groups.

Chairs are arranged in a circle or semicircle and the program starts when the leader asks a group member to report on his or her situation. This procedure continues to the end of the program by which time all caregivers have had a chance to introduce themselves, explain their relationship to the patient under their care, update the group on their current situation, and to make any statement or ask questions. This helps to keep our acquaintance alive and our knowledge up to date on each group member's current situation. This procedure creates a secure and non-threatening environment and a group camaraderie in which all feel free to vent their emotions, share their experiences, and even to express their humor without fear of being misunderstood. We become aware that we are all in the same situation struggling with common problems. There is no better place to find new, understanding, and empathetic friends. There is no better place to learn about the effects of Alzheimer's on its victims and their caregivers, and to find and exchange caregiving techniques. Within the safe structure of the group, caregivers find the moral support they need to carry their burden and escape becoming secondary victims.

Finding Humor in the Midst of Tragedy

All of us who are Alzheimer caregivers know, or should know, the value of humor in the tragic situation through which we are living. "There is little else that will make a person feel as good as a good laugh," says Anisman-Saltman, humorist and professor at Southern Connecticut State University. "Laughing," she says, "unites us with everybody else who's laughing, so it is impossible to feel lonely when you are laughing in a group of people."

Reader's Digest has a section in every issue called, "Laughter, the Best Medicine." Josh Billings said, "There ain't much fun in medicine, but there's a heck of a lot of medicine in fun." Fredrich Nietzsche said, "The most acutely suffering animal on earth invented laughter." The late Norman Cousins, author of *Anatomy of an Illness* and more recently *Head First,* who was noted for his belief in the curative value of humor, reports "there is mounting scientific evidence that laughter and festivity can help combat serious illness."

There are some who say that humor is appropriate anywhere and on all occasions. I recently heard a humorous story about what might be considered the most inappropriate of all occasions—a funeral—and it was introduced by the deceased herself. She had been a lawyer who was noted for her humor. She wrote her own obituary, had it tape-recorded, and asked her minister to play it at her funeral. The mourners were astounded when the first words were, "Well, here I am, just as dead as a doorknob." It was reported that the remainder of the tape was so filled with humor that some were "in stitches" by the end of the recording.

I have heard it said by some people, who have never attended one of our meetings, that all we do is cry about our problems. I do not deny that there is some "crying on shoulders," but I have seen much more laughing than crying in our meetings. We do not laugh at the victims of Alzheimer's, but at the funny things they say and do. To bear our burdens, it helps to find humor in the tragedy we see.

The Covered-Dish Party

One support group I attended had a "covered-dish social," each Christmas, during which there was no mention of Alzheimer's or of our caregiving problems. Each family caregiver brought a covered dish of his or her choice and we enjoyed some very well-balanced meals, albeit they were a little heavy on the desserts! These socials were the most joyous meetings of the year. We ate, talked and laughed in an atmosphere of good fellowship. It was impossible to feel tense, lonely, or socially isolated at these events.

We not only found good food in the covered dishes and warm fellowship, but we also found laughter as we traded jokes and told funny anecdotes about ourselves and each other. A festive evening, spent among good friends, with good food and hearty laughter is just right for what ails us Alzheimer's caregivers. The hours I spent with the support groups provided me with more friendship, more moral support, and a greater psychosocial lift than an equal amount of time spent anywhere else, doing anything else.

The Alzheimer's support group is a lighthouse of help and hope where caregivers can meet empathetic friends who are walking in similar shoes; where they can express feelings, share experiences, lose the sense of aloneness, and have their hopes renewed. ⊹

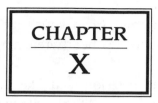

CHAPTER
X

THE NURSING HOME DECISION

An Agonizing and Heartbreaking Experience

The decision to put a loved one in a nursing home is never an easy one, whether made by the husband, wife, daughter, or some other relative. It is likely to be the most painful and difficult decision of one's life. It is seldom a clear-cut choice between what is perceived to be good and bad, but rather a choice between the lesser of two evils. Often it is not a matter of choice, but a necessity. That, however, does not necessarily lessen the pain.

A number of things may affect the difficulty of making such a decision and the severity of the emotional pain which follows. One's past experience with nursing homes and how one feels about them may be an important factor. The relationship of the decision-maker to the patient — husband, wife, father, mother, or other relative — is also important. Some nursing home personnel have expressed the opinion that it is more difficult for a husband than for any other relative. It has been said that, in our culture, the husband feels that, come what may, he must keep his wife at home and under his care, lest others think he no longer loves her. There is no way of knowing how much truth, if any, there is in this opinion but, speaking as a husband in a long and happy marriage, I can vouch for the fact that it has been the most agonizing, heartwrenching, and guilt-ridden decision of my life.

The nursing home decision is unlike the instinctive action which one would make in a life-threatening situations. If Bess were suddenly caught in a burning building, I would risk my life to save her without thinking of the consequences.. If she were in water and in danger of drowning, I would respond in the same way. The nursing home decision, however, is not a response to an immediate, life-threatening situation. There is time to think, time for an argument between the brain and the heart, time for reason versus feelings.

Unfortunately, my decision to place Bess in a nursing home was related to and influenced by an impending similar decision for her sister Mamie. Mamie had come under the care of me and my daughter, Estelle. The dementia had moved more rapidly in her than in Bess, and we decided that she would also have to be placed in a nursing home within a few months. Because of her financial condition, she would have to go on Medicaid, and we had discovered that all nursing homes had long waiting lists of Medicaid applicants. It was uncertain whether a vacancy would be available by the time she needed to go. In that case, one of us might have to take her into our home. For the sake of Bess, Mamie, and Estelle, it was important that I survive in good health and stay out of a nursing home myself.

A number of other factors entered into my struggle to make a decision. Bess and I had lived together so long that we had, in a sense, become a part of each other. Leaving her in the nursing home was like tearing us apart. We lost a part of ourselves which can never be restored; there were wounds that will never heal. Bess had lost much of her memory, but her memory of me and home had survived. She had lost her sense of self-reliance, and the only sources of security she knew were me and our home. To deny her that security was like taking a security blanket from a child. To leave her in a strange place among sick, handicapped people whom she had never seen would be a terrible emotional shock to her. She still had the capacity to suffer from such an experience.

I knew Bess well enough and had learned through caring for her at home and through her experience at ACTO that she had certain special needs which no nursing home, to my knowledge, was fully prepared to meet. Her needs were not primarily skilled nursing care, but recreational and social programs. I knew also that the recreational and social programs and staff of the nursing homes were inadequate for her needs. Why, then, did I put her there? Simply, I knew of no better place. My fears were that she would not accept the nursing home, nor would she be able to adjust to an institutional environment. And in that case, both the nursing home and I would have problems. As we shall see later, my fears were correct.

I found some help in Doug Manning's little book, *When Love Gets Tough*. According to his view, I had reached the point in my relationship with Bess where love does not mean doing what she wants to do or what I want to do; but, rather, it means doing what seems to be best for both of us. I had just about reached the end of my coping ability at home. Keeping her at home and trying to care for her would have destroyed me sooner or later. Despite my seeming selfishness, I realized that I must, for her sake and mine, save myself.

I finally found some comfort in the great Christian principle — "Do unto others as you would have them do unto you." I asked myself, if the situation were reversed and Bess were making this decision for me, would I want her to do as I was doing to her? My answer was yes; my brain had won over my heart.

The First Night in the Beginning of a New Life for Me

When I returned from the nursing home, I was stricken with sorrow for Bess, with grief from my loss of her, and with guilt for placing her there. My thoughts turned to the new kind of life I now faced. This was the end of our long marital relationship, but not the end of our marriage and love. It would be a life of loneliness during the remaining years of my old age. As long as she survived, my life would be dominated by my concern for her well-being at the nursing home. It would be a very different kind of life, and I would have to find ways to deal with it. My emotions were such that I could not look at TV, I could not read, and I could not write; so I took a long walk and began to think about how I could deal with this new life.

It had been an emotionally exhausting day and, following the walk, I was tired enough to sleep without difficulty. Late in the night, however, I was awakened by a nightmare. I dreamed that someone was breaking into the house. I froze. I could not move; I could not speak. After a moment of paralyzing fright, I regained my ability to function and sat up in bed. I listened, but not a sound was audible from anywhere. Although I then realized that it was only a dream, my heart was pounding as if it had been a real break-in. As I recovered my senses, I realized that Bess' side of the bed was empty. She was gone, gone forever. She would never again sleep beside me, as she had for more than 50 years. Not only would there be an empty place in my bed, but an empty place in my home, at my table, at my side when I visited friends, and an empty place in my heart.

Bess's First Reaction to her New Home

On the day I took Bess to the nursing home, I kissed her goodbye and left her without complaint on her part. She was in the care of a nurse and did not realize what was happening, nor where she was.

On the following day, I made my first visit. Then I got her reactions. Although I did not get the anger which I had expected, her reaction was one of surprise, disappointment, and disbelief. "Why have you put me in this jail? Why have you put me here among these crazies? This is the most awful place I have ever been. If you don't take me home, I will kill myself." Although she had never cursed or accused me of trying to get rid of her, she did say many times, "There is nothing physically wrong with me. You could take me home if you wanted to."

That day, I suffered the most traumatic experience of my life, and I left the nursing home a changed man. I felt like a broken-hearted child who had the urge to weep uncontrollably, but I could not do that. Why did a long and happy marriage and a meaningful old age have to end in such a cruel tragedy? Why did I do this to her? Why didn't I try harder to keep her at home? How can I live with this? This is a cruel punishment, which she does not deserve.

Her reactions and my emotions cut short my first visit to the nursing home; I left there in tears, cursing all the way home. I was not cursing Bess, or the nursing home, but the fate that had befallen us, the disease that was robbing her of her mind; I was cursing to keep from crying. I had never formed the habit of cursing and using profanity, but my inhibition was broken, and I found it the only way to express my feelings. More than once, I have left the nursing home in tears, not cursing audibly, but only in my thinking. This provided the relief I needed and often served as a convenient and effective coping technique.

A Second Nursing Home Decision

Just six months after placing Bess in a nursing home, my daughter and I had to make another nursing-home decision.

Mamie's condition had deteriorated rapidly. As soon as we realized that she could no longer cook, or even boil water for coffee, we arranged for Meals On Wheels to bring her one meal per
day, five days a week. Even though Estelle and I bought ready-
cooked food for the other meals during the week and the weekend, we soon began finding spoiled meats in her clothes closet,
under her pillow, and in her chest of drawers. We feared that she
would poison herself by eating spoiled food.

Estelle and I were each making two or three 30-mile trips a
week to care for her. Since long-distance caring was too costly
and too time-consuming, and the risk of food poisoning too
great, our only solution was a nursing home.

Since Mamie could not finance herself in a nursing home, and
neither I nor any other relative could do it, we sought Medicaid
for her. We were fortunate to find a home very near Estelle
which accepted her. Since the home in which I had placed Bess
did not accept Medicaid patients, it was not possible to place
Mamie there. By that time, the relationship between Bess and
Mamie had deteriorated to the point where it would have been
unwise to put them together in the same home.

Since Mamie had neither a husband nor a home to remember,
she was able to make an adjustment somewhat more easily
than Bess. Some of the nurses declared her one of the "sweetest, most friendly, and best-behaved residents" of the home.

I have had the unusual responsibility of putting two loved
ones in nursing homes within a six-month period, and that is
enough for one lifetime. My sincere hope is that the good Lord
will spare me from having to spend my last days in one, and I
am sure that Estelle hopes He will spare her of having to make
a third such decision.

With Bess and Mamie in different nursing homes, Estelle and
I shared responsibilities for visiting and looking after the two. I

had primary responsibility for Bess, and Estelle took primary responsibility for Mamie. It took me 25 minutes to reach Bess from my home and 45 minutes to reach Mamie. On the other hand, Estelle could reach Mamie quicker than she could reach Bess. I visited Mamie, but less often than Bess, and Estelle visited her mother, but less often than she did Mamie. Under the circumstances, this seemed the best arrangement we could make. ✐

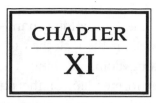

CHAPTER
XI

THE NURSING HOME EXPERIENCE

My Role in the Nursing Home

I knew that, as a husband and caregiver, I should, insofar as possible, continue a personal and meaningful relationship with Bess. She needed expressions of my love and care, and whatever I could do to help her adjust to her new life. I made an effort to establish a friendly and cooperative relationship with the nursing staff and aides under whose care she was. In that way, I felt I might be able to provide information about her which would be useful to the staff, and I needed their moral support. I had no wish to meddle with them in their work, but I needed the assurance that they were willing to listen to my suggestions concerning her care. I felt that her care should be a cooperative undertaking between her family and the nursing home, based on mutual respect. It has been my observation that many victims of Alzheimer's are simply dumped in nursing homes and are neglected or forgotten by their families.

Bess and Mary — a Companionship Based on Needs

Soon after Bess entered the first nursing home, I discovered that she and Mary, also a victim of Alzheimer's disease, were always together when I arrived for a visit. Often, I would find them walking down the hall holding hands, or in the room of one or the other, packing their clothes to go home. I seldom found them just sitting doing nothing. I knew nothing about Mary, nothing of her former life, or the nature of her trouble. Fortunately, I met her niece who was her sponsor in the nursing home and from her, I learned that Mary was widowed, that she had Alzheimer's, and that she had been born and reared in Kentucky. That information proved useful to me in trying to converse with Mary. She would talk about her life on the farm, about horses, the Kentucky Derby, and the weather in Kentucky. She would often comment on the local weather, saying, "It's a beautiful day," when it was really dark, cloudy, and threatening rain. To Mary, it was always a beautiful day. I also learned that she had been a legal secretary and could still take shorthand. I once tested her by dictating a letter and then having her read it back to me. She did it perfectly, but she could not have composed a letter of her own volition. This is an interesting and common occurrence with Alzheimer's patients. They often retain some former skill, which can be reactivated with stimulation from someone else. I soon decided that Mary must have been a sociable type of person, just as Bess had been. She was always kind, gracious, and polite to me. "Thank you so much for coming to see us. It was kind of you. If I had known you were coming, I would have cooked dinner." Often, when I announced that I had to leave, she would say, "If you will stay and have dinner with us, I will go to the kitchen and prepare it." I could carry on some kind of limited conversation with Mary, but not with Bess. It was difficult to separate them. If I did so, Bess would often ask, "Where is Mamie?" confusing Mary with her sister. Since they were so close, and Mary enjoyed my presence, I decided we would form a threesome, and I would try to find something the three of us could do together to bring pleasure into their lives.

Somehow, Bess and Mary had met, and found that they could relate to each other, and that the presence of the other satisfied their needs for the human touch and a social relationship. That companionship served a very great need in each of them for a warm social relationship and I was happy to see it.

Their relationship, however, was not always a peaceful one. On a few occasions, I saw them childishly quarreling, tugging, and fighting over a piece of clothing, each claiming it as her own. In their actions and arguments, they often reminded me of two little sisters in 80-year-old bodies. Each one's name was on her own clothing, but they never thought to look for it. I never saw them strike each other any more vigorously than tapping each other on the forearm, but I was told that their fights did become more violent. I could see the evidence in bruises on Bess's arms and hands. On one visit, as I went looking for them, I heard Bess talking very loudly and knew she was angry. I found them in the sitting room with most of the other residents. When Bess saw me, she came hurriedly to me saying, "Thank goodness you have come. That woman is driving me crazy." Then she said to Mary, "My husband is here. If you don't shut up, he will take care of you." That day, we did not form a threesome. I took Bess to her room, where we spent about an hour. When we came out, we passed by the sitting room, where Bess saw Mary and waved to her. Mary waved back and hurried to us, and the two hugged and kissed as if they had not seen each other in six months.

Since Bess was having difficulty with her roommates and with other residents, I thought it might be a good idea to place Bess and Mary in a room together. Although I had not suggested it, on one visit, a nurse asked if I would object to putting them together in the same room. On the contrary, I approved of the idea. Mary was in a room with three beds and two roommates.

Since that room was less costly than a private room or a semi-private one, it was much in demand, and we had to wait for a vacancy to occur. Eventually, one did occur, and Bess was moved in with Mary and a third person. I was sure this would be pleasing to both Bess and Mary, and I hoped there would be no difficulty with the other roommate. It was not long, however, before this third roommate was moved. The woman who replaced her was bedridden and unable to talk. I never knew who started it or why but, one weekend Bess and Mary beat up on their new roommate. As a result, she was moved out, and the two were left alone in the room with three beds. Bess and Mary remained without a third roommate for about three months. Except for little quarrels over clothing, they got along splendidly. Eventually, the nursing home had an applicant for the space, and I was informed that they would have to fill the vacant bed. For some reason, I never knew why, Bess was moved out to another room. Again, the nursing staff was faced with the problem of finding a roommate with whom Bess was compatible.

The friendship between Bess and Mary eased my leave-takings from the nursing home. Bess always wanted me to stay with her, or to take her home. She might say, "You're not going to leave me here alone, are you?" I would then ask Mary, "May Bess spend the night with you?" Mary was always happy to have her do so although they might not be rooming together at the time. On occasion, Mary might say, "If you will stay with us, I will go prepare dinner, and you can eat with us." I would say, "If you two will prepare dinner for me tomorrow, I will come to eat with you." Mary would then ask, "What do you like to eat?" We would orally prepare a menu, from soup to nuts, and I would say, "Now, don't forget; I will be here." They, of course, would forget before I got out of the building. Some people may call this strategy outright lying, but caregivers refer to it as "creative thinking."

Whatever one may call it, it worked for me in many situations and I felt that the end justified the means. I often had to withhold the truth from Bess about a number of things and to distance myself from her. She lost her sister to Alzheimer's and a brother to Parkinson's Disease during her days in the nursing home, but I didn't tell her. Hiding this information from her left me with a sense of guilt, and I was never able to evade the truth with a clear conscience. My relationship with her in the nursing home often became a sham and this was extremely difficult for me to cope with.

Making my Visits Meaningful and Enjoyable

After Bess entered the nursing home, I soon discovered that, if my visits were to be worthwhile, I would have to find something we could do together. What do you do when there is nothing you can talk about except home? I first tried entertaining Bess by taking in a box of old family photographs, but Bess quickly lost interest in looking at those, and they were meaningless to Mary. I then took in Bess' old college annual, and we tried looking through it, but that did not work either. I tried taking her for short outings and we would stop off and have an ice-cream sandwich. Bess enjoyed that; Mary wanted to go, too, but the nurses could not allow it. The nursing staff granted my request to take Bess back to the ACTO Center every Thursday. There, Bess participated in the program, enjoyed it, and found a few hours of meaningful life once each week. That led me to believe that an ACTO program, either in the nursing home, or a convenient distance from it, would work very well. But there was little response to that idea. Although Mary wanted to go with us, and would have participated in the program, I could not take her. I continued taking Bess, though, until I withdrew her from that home.

The most successful activity I found was an old marble-and-dice game called "Aggravation," which Bess and I used to play with our friends. Two to six people could play. Each player is given one die and four marbles of different colors. The object is to move the player's marbles around a board more quickly than any other player. A toss of the die determines how many places one may move the marble. Some thought and imagination, as well as luck, were required to win. Bess remembered the rules very well, but to keep the game going without argument, I often had to change marbles with her in the middle of the game. She would forget the color of the marbles with which she had started, and, since she often forgot the rules, we would play by her rules. Mary told me that she had never played the game, and I soon discovered she was unable to learn. She did not know whether she should toss the marble or the die. Once she had tossed her die, she did not know how many places to move; I would end up virtually having to play the entire game for her. Surprisingly, she never objected to my helping and never lost interest in the game. Bess, however, often became impatient with Mary and called her dumb or crazy, to which Mary never responded. I often cheated on their behalves, so that one or the other of them would win, thus maintaining each one's sense of self-worth. Then we would clap our hands, and I would praise the winner. The interest of Alzheimer's patients is usually very short-term, and it is difficult to maintain their interest in anything for more than a short period of time. It was amazing to me that both of them could play Aggravation for an hour and a half without losing interest. When Mary began to lose interest, she would say, "It is about time for dinner. You folks play, while I go and prepare dinner." Once, just before I left, Mary turned to Bess and asked, "What do we do now?" Bess said sarcastically, "Just sit and look at each other." Mary said, "Oh horrors. I can't think of anything worse."

Those statements were not only amusing, but tragic, indicating how they abhorred having nothing more to do than sit and look at each other or stare at the bare walls. That is often the kind of miserable life we condemn them to when we place them in a nursing home. That is why I felt guilty and grieved for Bess. That is also one reason why I continued to go to the nursing home regularly and tried to help her find some meaning in her life.

One may ask, how can an 85-year old man go to a nursing home and play a silly game with two senile and childish 80-year-old women, and still preserve his own sanity? I did it for a number of reasons: I loved Bess, and it hurt me to see her suffering from meaningless inactivity and from her longing for home and me. I went because I had found a simple little game which the three of us could play together to provide them an hour of pleasurable activity and social interaction. I did it to prove that it is possible to find a way to improve the quality of life for many of these people, who have nothing better to do for most of the day than to stare at the bare walls or at each other.

Finding Humor in the Nursing Home

Putting Bess in a nursing home and visiting her was no laughing matter. The sights I saw, the sounds I heard, the odors I smelled, and the emotions I felt were more conducive to sorrow, grief, and depression than to laughter. It is not an environment in which one would expect to find humor. Humorous incidents in this situation are few and far between, and often unexpected. If I was to endure the depressing emotions which bore down on me, I had to find humor to preserve my emotional stability. Robert Fulghum says, "Laughter is the only cure for grief." Fortunately, I have been able to find a few occasions for laughter which, although they have not cured me, have certainly given me relief.

Although I was not a party to the following story, I might well have been. I am told of a minister who was visiting a nursing home, going from one resident to the other, shaking hands and talking to those confined to wheelchairs. He noticed that one woman kept staring at him. When he reached her, he asked, "Have we met somewhere before?" She said, "No." He said, "You kept looking at me. I thought perhaps we had met, and I had forgotten." She said, "No, I just think you look like my second husband." He asked, "How many times have you been married?" She replied, "Once."

People in nursing homes are hungry for the human touch. Many of them will reach out to touch and kiss the hand of a friendly person. A lady in a wheelchair reached for my hand as I walked past her in the hall. She pulled it to her lips, kissed it, and asked, "Is everything paid for?" I assured her it was, and she released my hand. Another reached out for my hand and said, "Your hand is cold." I squeezed her hand slightly, and she said, "There. That is better." As Bess and I were walking down the hall one day, we passed a woman in a wheelchair. She was physically crippled but, apparently, there was nothing wrong with her mind. She was one of the few residents with whom I could carry on an intelligent conversation, but she had, at times, a rather cruel sense of humor. She liked to tease Bess, and that probably led to what had happened a few days before. As we passed her, she said to me, "Bess pulled my hair the other day." I had already heard about the incident.

After Bess was confined to a wheelchair, I entered a long hall leading to her room, and I saw her and the woman whose hair she had pulled sitting across the hall from each other. Bess said, "There comes my husband," and the woman said, "No, that's my husband." When I reached them, Bess was angry, and the woman was laughing. I kissed Bess and said, "There, that proves

100

whose husband I am." The woman kept up the ruse, however, and again said, "No." I wondered how much pain these people suffered from one anothers' attempts to retain their individualism, to retain something of their own personalities, even if at the expense of another.

Although Bess was a much larger and taller person than Mary, they often wore each other's clothing. On one visit, I found them walking down the hall holding hands. Bess was wearing a pair of Mary's pants, which were too small and too short. Over the pants, she had on Mary's dress and, over that, she wore Mary's jacket. Mary was wearing a pair of Bess' pants, which were too long and too large. She had on a blouse which belonged to Bess and, over that, she wore a very large, long sweater, which I had never seen before. It hung halfway to her knees. That was a laughable sight; I have often wished that I had a picture of it.

Alzheimer's robbed Bess of her best, most human and most distinguishing traits as an individual—her ability to remember, to think, to understand, to converse, and to socialize with other people. Along with those losses went her self-initiative and her self-esteem. In short, she lost her "self," the unique and wonderful person she used to be. One part of herself, however, she did not lose, until the very last, and that was her sense of humor. I was surprised that much of the humor I experienced in the nursing home came from Bess herself, as she used to be. The nurses and the aides in the nursing home also saw some of it. One day, while she was in the first nursing home, I took her by the nursing station, and she said to the nurse, "Why don't you let me go home with my husband? I am no good here. All I do is take up space." The nurse laughed and, since I was having some difficulty getting away to go home, I asked her if Bess might spend the night with her. She said, "Sure. I will be happy to have her." I then left without difficulty. Another day, while she was in the second home, the doctor came to examine her, and when he said, "Let me examine your heart," Bess said, "Oh, it's okay; they just gave me a new one yesterday."

The last expression of humor in Bess was about three weeks before she died. One Sunday after lunch, I wheeled her down to the lobby, as usual, where there was a rack full of magazines, some of which she had subscribed to and read before Alzheimer's robbed her of the ability to read. I had discovered that if I gave her a magazine, she would sit and turn through it, page after page, looking at pictures and reading the titles of articles. She would never stop to read anything other than the titles. She would often hold the magazine out before me and point to a picture or a title she wanted me to see. I would make some comment about it, and she would continue turning and looking and, as long as I sat by her side, she seemed content. One day, she held the magazine out in front of me and pointed to the title of an article she wanted me to see. It read, "How To Have An Affair With Your Husband." I almost jumped out of the chair and said, "Honey, if you will read it and learn how, I will take it home." That was a good one to end up with, and I will never forget it.

Withdrawing Bess from the Nursing Home

Bess had been in the nursing home for a little more than two years and had been a problem for the staff and administration for most of that period. It had been impossible to find her another compatible roommate. Since Mary had become less active and slept for much of the afternoon. Bess was alone for most of the time, and could find no one to whom she could relate. She became bored to death, with nothing to do and no meaningful social relationship. Her hearing had become so poor that she could talk with very few people, and because of poor hearing, she began to talk very loudly and became verbally abusive, as well. She became bossy and demanding, and would often strike others for no reason. She was in rebellion against the situation in which she found herself and the people around her.

When I finally went to speak with the nursing home administrator, he told me that the State Department of Human Resources was demanding to know what he was going to do about her. If she struck another person, he would be in serious trouble with the Department. In that case, it would be necessary to sedate her heavily so that she would be unable to continue striking people. Since I did not want to see her under such sedation, I decided to withdraw her from the home.

I was faced with another difficult problem. I had taken her to the nursing home because I could not cope with her at home. After two years in the nursing home, they could no longer manage her. What should I do with her now? The best place I had found for her was the ACTO Daycare Center, but it was limited to one day per week. She needed more than one day a week of that kind of care, and I needed more than one day of relief. I had placed her at an Alzheimer's daycare center, but she simply refused to stay there. I found another daycenter which had a vacancy one day per week, but she liked it even less. Since two days of respite care a week were not enough, I knew that, sooner or later, as her disease progressed, I would have to return her to a nursing home.

Some of my friends had reported good results from taking a mother or father to a psychiatric clinic and suggested I try it. I knew the only thing the clinic could do would be to sedate her, so she could be managed. I had no faith in that, and I did not want to keep her under permanent sedation. I felt that she could be managed through the right kind of recreational activities and social program, the kind I had discovered at ACTO. After three weeks with her at home, and despite my doubts and misgivings, I was ready to try anything that had any chance of success. It was under those circumstances that I decided to try the clinic. ∽

CHAPTER
XII

THE CLINIC & THE SECOND NURSING HOME

I applied to a Clinic, and Estelle and I made the necessary preparations for entering Bess. When we arrived, she walked in without assistance. We went through the process of admission, supplied the necessary background information, and were shown to her room. There we met the doctor, his assistant, two nurses, and two medical students. The doctor asked a few questions of me and of Bess, then told us it required about 12 days for the necessary examinations to find the proper medical treatment for her condition. Estelle and I then left, with Bess protesting. We promised to return the next day.

The following day, we found Bess in a wheelchair and under restraint, begging us to take her home. We also noticed that she no longer had a roommate, but was alone. Those two things indicated to me that they were having difficulty with her, but I asked no questions. I hoped that the restraint would be temporary. That afternoon, Estelle received a telephone call from the clinic and was told that it would be necessary for Bess to have personal care 24 hours a day. That was a shocking revelation to me since she had never needed that kind of care at the nursing home. I had assumed that the clinic had the nurses and staff required to provide the necessary care. Personal care would be a considerable extra cost and would not be included in what I was already paying the clinic for her care. I doubted that either Medicare or my insurance would pay any part of that extra cost. I now know that I should have withdrawn her, that very moment, from the clinic. Instead, we asked the clinic to secure the necessary personal care. Surely, this 24-hour-a-day care would be temporary.

When we returned to the clinic the next day, we found Bess under personal care and heavily sedated. She could not walk without assistance; she could not get into nor out of the bed to go to the bathroom; she could not safely be left alone; and she was not only physically helpless, but senseless, as well. She begged us to take her home, saying, "They are preparing to kill me here." She remained under 24-hour personal care and, in that condition, for the remaining 11 days in the clinic. That was the most horrible emotional experience of my life and I came nearer then to a complete emotional breakdown than I have ever been.

What about the financial costs? I was paying the clinic $655.00 per day for room, board and nursing care. The personal care was an extra $180.00 per day, which brought my daily costs to $835.00. That was a terrible price to pay for a failed experiment. She was, in fact, in worse condition when we removed her than when we entered her. That, however, was not the end of this experience.

When we removed Bess from the clinic, she had to be carried out in a wheelchair and lifted into the car. When we arrived home, two men carried her into the house and put her to bed. Estelle spent the night with us. Since we did not, at the time, have a guardrail to keep her from falling out of bed, we took turns checking on her about every fifteen minutes. Late in the night, when we were ready to go to bed, I found her on the floor. She had not called, but had tried to go to the bathroom and had fallen on the floor beside the bed. Fortunately, there was a carpet on the floor, and she was not hurt. She weighed about 175 pounds, dead weight, and she was completely unable to help Estelle and me to get her off the floor. In our efforts to get her up, I brought on an old lower-back problem, which left me helpless. We called the County Medical Emergency Unit to get her to the bathroom and back to bed. For five days, I had to have personal care 24-hours a day, at a cost of $240.00 per day. I was not only physically broken, I was also emotionally exhausted and was rapidly going bankrupt.

Another Nursing Home Decision

When we brought Bess home from the clinic, we were given instructions about reducing her medication. Five days after she returned home, she could walk again, but still needed some assistance in getting into and out of bed and going to the bathroom. Estelle and I both realized that the only thing to do was to return her to a nursing home. The only choice was to decide whether we should return her to the one from which I had withdrawn her, or find another suitable one. We were certain that her problem of adjustment had not been solved, but thought that a change might improve her chances. We investigated one I had visited earlier. From all appearances, it was as good as the one from which I had withdrawn her. I did not, however, find any better activities or social programs than I had found in the previous home.

We talked at length with the head nurse and told her about the problems Bess had at the previous home and our experience with the clinic. She felt that she and her staff had a good record of managing patients with similar problems. She said that sedation might become necessary, but promised not to sedate her to the point of helplessness. It so happened that a vacancy existed in a room with two vacant beds, directly across the hall from the nursing station. Bess would be alone, for awhile, at least. We accepted it, and moved her in immediately.

By that time, Bess was back on her feet and able to walk without assistance, to feed herself, and to clothe herself. I was deeply concerned about the possibility of her getting out and into the street because the front door of the nursing home was within 100 feet of a very heavily traveled street. Bess soon found her way to the door and out, but they kept a watch on her and prevented her from getting to the street. As long as she could walk, she continued her efforts to escape the nursing home, and I frequently found her under mild sedation when I went to lunch with her twice a week.

For about three months, Bess remained the only person in her room and, if there were any serious incidents of combativeness, I was not informed about them. I found the aides at the second home to be better-trained, more sociable, and more able to deal with her and that made a difference. Bess was finally given a roommate, a black woman. If there were any conflicts or other problems with her roommate, I was not told of them. After about a year, Bess was placed in a room with three roommates. There were no problems in that situation although Bess never found another person like Mary with whom she could relate so well. The only time she associated with her roommates was at bedtime. There was simply no meaningful social relationship with them; her socializing was mostly with the aides and the nurses. When I went to have lunch with Bess, I most often found her sitting with another Alzheimer's patient who could not talk loud enough for Bess to understand her. The only socializing they did was just sit together. There were five or six people there who were not victims of Alzheimer's, but rather had physical difficulties. They seemed to like Bess, would often talk with her, and that had some value for her.

An interesting feature of the second nursing home was the eating arrangement for those visiting a loved one. On one side of the diningroom, two tables were arranged together, so as to accommodate six people. I had lunch with Bess twice a week, and we ate at that table with others who were visiting residents. This led to some conversation, but Bess never participated unless others spoke to her; then, she would always reply.

Five months after Bess entered the nursing home, she developed pneumonia. The nursing staff decided to keep her in the nursing home rather than send her to the hospital, and she probably received better care there. Since her room was located directly across the hall from the nursing station, she was within ten feet of the nurses all day. A home X-ray was available at all times, and the doctor saw her frequently. I was pleased by the way she was cared for by the aides. For awhile, she was in very serious condition, and I feared that she would not recover. She was confined to bed for a month and lost her ability to walk; after that, she was confined to a wheelchair, and never walked again. She became completely urinary incontinent; she often had difficulty breathing, and needed medication.

Words of Love that Broke my Heart

Throughout her stay in the nursing home, Bess continued to ask me to take her home. She would often say, "You could take me home if you wanted to." She would also say, "The two things I want most in the world are you and home." It hurt that I had to deny her both. I always kissed her when I left and, if I said, "I love you," she would say, "I love you too, more than you will ever know." How do you cope with such words?

I once arranged for an aide to accompany us, so that I could take her home for lunch, which I had already prepared. As I rolled her into the livingroom, I asked, "Do you know where you are?" She said, "No," but, pointing to an enlarged picture of her favorite grandmother, she said, "That's grandma's picture." I showed her a number of needlecraft pictures that she herself had made, but she could not recall having made a single one of them. After lunch, she said, "Let's go home," and we returned to the nursing home. She no longer knew home when she got there, but she still had a memory of home that never left her. Up until the night she died, she was still asking to go home.

The years she spent in the nursing homes were horrible years for me. My knowledge of her, my empathy and compassion, enabled me to feel and share her sufferings—idleness, boredom, confusion, fear, and social isolation—a kind of hell on earth. My sorrow, my frustrations, and my feelings of helplessness threatened to overcome me. To preserve my own physical, mental, and emotional well-being, I had to find ways to cope with those feelings.

I often awoke in the middle of the night, with my mind racing like a car on the race track, and it was impossible to go to sleep again. Since I could not just lie there and roll and tumble, I had to do something. I tried taking my regular morning exercise, but that did not help. I tried counting sheep; counting from 1 to 100; counting the number of states in our union; and finally, counting the countries, by name, from Mexico through Central and South America. That did not slow me down. The only solution was to get up and get busy — to read, write, or go to the kitchen to bake breads or cakes. Following that, I ate an early breakfast, returned to bed, and got one to two hours additional sleep. There was no respite from my heavy burden. Her four years in the nursing homes were bitter years of disappointment, frustration, helplessness, and grief. Without the support of my family, my good neighbors, the Alzheimer's family support group, my exercise, and my writing, I could not have survived in good health. ↜

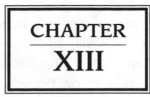

CHAPTER
XIII

SPECIAL CARE UNITS AND OTHER MODELS OF CARE

Although I had to place Bess in a nursing home, I knew this was not the ideal placement for her. I was convinced that there was a need for a better place to care for the victims of this cruel disease than the conventional nursing home. When Bess said, "Why did you put me in this jail? Why did you put me here with these crazies?" she expressed her feelings about being thrust into a strange and unfamiliar world with strangers who seemed to her to be crazy. How could I, a compassionate and loving husband, do this to my beloved wife and bear the burden? That became my most difficult problem.

Essential Features of A New Model of Care

Although there is an ever growing number of dementia patients who are in need of better facilities, there was at that time little information on the subject. The few daycare centers which were being established were unable to meet the patients' needs. For the most part, we were putting our loved ones in totally inappropriate and unqualified nursing homes, in some cases the worst sort of place. There they lived out their remaining years in inactivity, boredom, and social isolation. Clearly a new model of care was needed to help patients find a better life, a life of meaning, self-worth, and dignity so as to escape idleness, boredom, and social isolation. The special care units now proliferating around the country have the following features:

- **A SEPARATE UNIT, EITHER IN OR OUTSIDE THE NURSING HOME.** Since their primary needs are different, people with Alzheimer's disease require a separate unit designed and operated to meet their special needs. To house them with others who do not have a similar problem makes stress for both, especially for the former.

- **A HOMELIKE ENVIRONMENT.** In so far as possible, each patient should be able to lead a normal life, do the familiar things he or she used to do and feel more at home than in the conventional nursing home. It is very unwise to put Alzheimer's patients in a strange and unfamiliar place with people they do not understand and with whom they cannot find a meaningful social relationship. The staff members should be able to discover the special needs and surviving capabilities of each patient and then find ways to use those abilities to satisfy their needs. The staff's role involves more than caregiving. It involves enabling, the ability to provide the initiative and guidance to **enable** the patient to use his or her surviving mental and physical abilities. They should be able to fit into the role of kind, loving friends who can help ward off social isolation and help people to have a sense of belonging.

- **RECREATIONAL ACTIVITIES, BOTH MENTAL AND PHYSICAL.** We all have an innate need to do things, to take care of our individual needs, to be useful and independent. To lose those capacities reduces our humanness and leads to frustration and confusion. To find meaning in their lives these people, like little children, need help in relearning to do what they once did to find meaning and a sense of worth. Such activities should be individualized in order to fit the special needs of each individual.

Those features, drawn from my personal experiences, observations and reading are the unique qualities of a successful caring program for people with Alzheimer's. We need more experimentation, testing, and scientific evaluation to determine the truth. Can we do it? Can we afford it? How long will our humanness, our concepts and caring natures permit us to continue to accept the dehumanizing consequences of not doing it?

In 1992, The National Institute on Aging (NIA) announced the award of $2.25 million for research on the effectiveness and costs of special care units in nursing homes for people with Alzheimer's disease. The Special Care Units Initiative funded nine coordinated projects to evaluate the impact of these programs on people with Alzheimer's disease, their families, and nursing home staff.

What if Bess had been in a Special Care Unit?

Had Bess been in a special care unit such as I have described, she would not have forgotten about her longings for home and for me, but they would have been reduced to a minimum. She would have been in a more homelike environment, which was less like what she called "a jail." She would have been under the care of trained people who knew how to promote the initiative and provide the leadership which she needed and to whom she could relate socially. She would have found recreational activities and meaningful social interactions to keep her hands and mind busy. The staff would have been able to help her resume, insofar as possible, the normal activities and social roles which had been so much a part of her former life. She would have gained a sense of belonging, which would have reduced her homesickness. It would have relieved her of boredom, social isolation, loneliness, and stress which were the source of her sufferings in the nursing home. She could have had a better life, a life more full of meaning, worth, and joy, for as long as possible, until the time of her death. What about me, her caregiver? I would have found relief from knowing that she was in the friendly hands of people who knew her special needs and were able to provide the initiative and guidance to help her satisfy those needs. I would have felt relieved that I had done my best to find her a better life.

Examples of Special Care Units

A few nursing homes around the country are experimenting with special units for Alzheimer's patients. I have made no effort to determine the number, to compare them, or to evaluate them. I have, however, selected three which seem to represent the basic features of this emerging model of care.

Christian City

Christian City, near Atlanta, Georgia, operates a special Alzheimer's unit which provides a home for patients who have been diagnosed with dementia. The unit provides a secure and homelike environment with open doors leading to a fenced-in outer area. Live-in caregivers are trained to deal with Alzheimer patients and to provide love and companionship. One purpose of the unit is to assist patients and challenge them to use their surviving capabilities to reach their maximum potential. The unit maintains a program of varied activities, both inside and outside, to keep the patients active mentally and physically. Depending on the season of the year and the weather, the outside program consists of daily trips, picnicking, fishing, swimming, sightseeing, and participating in community activities. They encourage interaction between staff, patients, and families. Medical and nursing services are provided by visiting doctors and nurses.

Logan Hall

A second special unit approach is Logan Hall, located in Logan Hall Green Hills Center at West Liberty, Ohio. Logan Hall was established in 1980 as a "Special Care Area" for Alzheimer's patients. At that time there was little precedent for a separate unit and a special care program. In a recent letter, the administrator says that Logan Hall is "considered by experts such as Nancy Mace to be one of the more successful units in the country". The idea of a separate unit grew out of concern for the "quality of life for some of the patients... those who suffered from dementia, and their roommates or neighbors, who were affected by their special problems". The conclusion was that it would be better to separate the Alzheimer's patients from the others and prepare a special care program in a separate unit. Two basic factors determined the nature of the new unit: a homelike environment and a specially trained staff to operate the program. Their major goal is to preserve each resident's "dignity and self-worth, with emphasis on providing a routine and calm environment and a consistent daily pattern". Since each resident has different needs and stages, the program is individualized to meet their needs. Every day, residents participate in physical activities, such as tossing a ball, walking, and exercising. They sing hymns and old favorite songs, and those who wish may work at simple puzzles, games, or crafts. Men may sand parts of toys prepared by other residents to be given to the Child Center or to be sold to the public. Women may crochet, knit, cut, or sew quilt patches. In the summer, residents plant and grow flowers and vegetables. The women may help with the preparation of meals, setting the table, and cleaning up after meals. Twice each week, there is interaction with the children of the Child Center which is a part of the complex of Green Hills Center. One day the residents of Logan Hall visit the Child Center and another day the children visit Logan Hall. A monthly picnic includes the families of the residents. The social workers relate closely with the families and play a supportive role.

The staff at Logan Hall and the physicians involved believe that "it provides a setting where a certain quality of life can be maintained in spite of decreasing functions. A comfortable, familiar place, well-trained staff offering warmth and acceptance to both residents and families, and individualized activities that provide the proper amount and kind of stimulation — these are the ingredients most important for a therapeutic situation which preserves each person's identity and optimal functioning, and creates a truly special home."

Wesley Hall

A third example of the special unit approach is Wesley Hall, located in the Chelsea United Methodist Retirement Home at Chelsea, Michigan. The unit was designed and furnished to create a warm homelike environment. It is provided with equipment and materials to enable residents to live normal lives insofar as possible. In training a special staff, the emphasis was on being an "enabler" rather than a "caregiver." They were trained to find and use the patients' surviving abilities for as long as possible. The emphasis is on looking for the residents' remaining strengths rather than focusing on their behavioral problems. The activities program is built on the former interests and abilities of the individual. Close family relationships are encouraged and potluck dinners play an important role in keeping alive this relationship.

In all these special programs, the key factor is a specially trained staff whose members function as "enablers" who create activities which enable patients to use their remaining strengths and abilities. Alzheimer's patients need activities which are within their limited abilities and they need help to engage in these activities. They need association with friendly people to give them a sense of belonging and of security. Special units can relieve the conventional nursing homes of problems they are not equipped to deal with and provide Alzheimer's patients a better life.

The Personal Care Home

The rapid increase in the number of aged people with dementia and the high cost of nursing home care has led to the establishment of personal care homes, owned and operated by private individuals. Under current state law in Georgia, a personal care home is permitted to house residents needing only some supervision with everyday routines, such as bathing and eating. A personal care resident must be coherent enough to perceive an emergency such as a fire and be physically able to respond.

At present, there are about 1,400 licensed personal care homes in Georgia, housing about 12,000 residents. The state estimates that hundreds of personal care homes are operating illegally without a license. The Department of Human Resources has only three people to keep track of all these homes and no full-time nurses or doctors to inspect them. It is well-known that many of these are housing Alzheimer's victims and they are operating outside the law. During the last five years, dozens of complaints have been made but officials simply look the other way. Judith Hageback, director of the Department of Human Resources' Office of Aging says, "It is a disaster just waiting to happen. And it's scary." We have one of the most rapidly growing small scale industries in the state, many of which are operating outside the law and housing a growing number of mentally disabled people such as Alzheimer's victims, yet we are paying little attention to it. Many caregivers in these homes do not have the qualifications to provide the kind of care which these people need. Those who are placing their loved one in personal care homes have no other place to put them. They have too much income to place them under Medicaid and not enough to place them in a nursing home.

The Atlanta Alzheimer's chapter has started a program, called **Partners in Care** which consults with homes and health agencies. It requires participants to meet new guidelines detailed by the National Alzheimer's Association. If it is to be successful, the state must provide qualified inspection and enforceable regulation. People who place an Alzheimer's patient in one of these personal care homes need to know the home is qualified to offer the kind of care which patients need. People will need to know that the patient is safe from abuse and that the home will do what it says it will do. The state must provide the inspection and regulation to see that each home is up to the standards set for them. No home should operate without first being licensed. ⊷

CHAPTER
XIV

Alzheimer's Awareness Programs

A Closer Look at Alzheimer's for Medical Students

Few aspiring physicians are aware of the problems faced by family members and health care providers in caring for patients with dementia. Traditional coursework usually doesn't address the emotional, physical, and financial stresses that patients and their caregivers experience.

Medical students at Emory University in Atlanta, Georgia, are exposed to these issues through the Alzheimer's Disease Awareness Program, organized by the Emory Alzheimer's Disease Center and the Atlanta Area Chapter of the Alzheimer's Association. The goal of this program is to sensitize students to these often neglected issues by providing them with a memorable experience during their early training. Second year medical students meet with caregivers and their affected family members at the patient's home, nursing home, or day care center. An average of 25 families volunteer each year to meet with small groups. Students not only meet the patients but also have the opportunity to ask the caregivers about the problems they've faced, their experiences with physicians and other health care professionals, and their sources of support. The students write a short summary of their impressions, while families receive a personalized letter of appreciation. For many students who have little "hands on" experience, this exposure remains a highlight of their medical training and, although the one-time visit takes at most an hour or two, the experience can have a lasting effect.

Many Alzheimer's caregivers, puzzled and worried by the unusual symptoms they are seeing in a loved one, have taken the patient to the doctor, looking for an answer, and have returned home disappointed and bewildered. They discovered the doctor had no answers. He knew no cause, no cure, and no effective means of treating the symptoms. There was no way to make a definitive diagnosis prior to death and autopsy. Unfortunately, caregivers left the doctor's office feeling that the doctor was not only lacking in knowledge about the disease, but also was lacking in concern, compassion or interest. Often, the doctor never mentioned Alzheimer's, but suggested as possible causes of the symptoms "hardening of the arteries," "senility," "senile dementia," or "organic brain syndrome." Such terms did not satisfy me, nor do they satisfy many other caregivers. Until recently, most family caregivers had never heard the term "Alzheimer's disease," but we knew we had a strange and difficult problem on our hands which was threatening our own emotional and physical well-being. The doctor did not seem to be aware of it; at least, he had said nothing about it, and had not mentioned any source of help, which caregivers desperately needed. I personally have had three instances in which I thought there was lack of empathy and understanding on the part of the doctors for what Bess and I were going through.

There is, no doubt, a problem here, but lest we be too harsh on the doctors, it should be said that not all caregivers have left doctor's offices with the feeling that he was lacking in concern about their problem. In some cases, they found empathy in a simple question asked by the doctor, "Well, how are you getting along?"

The seeming lack of knowledge and concern may be due to some gaps in the medical education of doctors. Awareness of Alzheimer's Disease is new, and not until the last two decades was it generally believed to be a disease of the aged. Since very little was known about it, the symptoms were thought to be a normal part of the aging process. There were not such large numbers of people afflicted by dementing symptoms as there are today. Since it was generally believed that the cause was merely old age, rather than a disease, it was a matter of little concern in the education of physicians. Although much scientific study and research had gone into efforts to find a cure for such killer diseases as heart attack and cancer, there had been no similar effort directed toward Alzheimer's disease.

The rapid extension of life has brought us many new health problems, one of which is the growing prevalence of a long-known but mysterious disease, now called Alzheimer's. We are slowly becoming aware of the devastating impact not only on its victims, but on their caregivers as well. In dealing with Alzheimer's, we must not forget the family caregivers. I like the advice given the doctors of Alzheimer's patients at the Brookdale Center of Aging in New York City: "Treat the patient as well as the disease; treat the caregiver as well as the patient."

In addition to classroom lectures, books, and medical school laboratories, there are three ways to gain a realistic awareness of Alzheimer's disease, its nature, its effects on the victim, and the problems it creates for the family caregiver. A caregiver needs to be a caregiver; to exchange experiences with other caregivers at a support group, or to observe the patient in a real-life situation. No other disease creates for the family quite the same kind of situation as Alzheimer's. Few doctors have had an opportunity to see the patient outside the office or nursing home. Some medical educators have conceived the idea that it would be a valuable part of their education if young medical students had an opportunity to observe Alzheimer's patients in real-life situations.

With Dr. Suzanne Mirra as director, The Emory University School of Medicine in Atlanta, Georgia, has established an Alzheimer's Awareness Program in which all second-year medical students are required to participate. The "goal is to expose medical students, early in their careers, to the problems of Alzheimer's disease for the patient and the caregiver." They want the students not only to see the victim of this disorder, but also to hear firsthand what the family's experiences have been.

Working through the local unit of the Alzheimer's Association, Dr. Mirra finds families in the community in which there is a victim of the disease, contacts the caregiver, explains the program, and asks if he or she would be interested in participating. If the response is positive, she sends a form to be filled out and returned, in which the caregiver lists a convenient place, time, and number of students desired for the meeting. The meeting place may be the home of the caregiver, a daycare center, or a nursing home. The program director then selects the students to attend the meeting and designates a leader of the group to contact the caregiver to make arrangements for the meeting.

Student Response

Bess and I participated in two programs, the first in the nursing home in 1988, and the second in our home, a year later. Five students came to the first meeting. I first met with the students alone, explained to them the beginning of Bess' symptoms, how they had affected me, and how I was trying to cope with them. I told them some specific instances of her memory loss, her changed behavior, her nagging, and her stubbornness about taking baths. I related some instances of her behavior in the nursing home and her inability to adjust to institutional living and to the other residents. I also pointed out to them a distinguishing feature of Alzheimer's disease, which I had observed in Bess; that is, it destroyed certain human qualities, such as memory, self-initiative, self-reliance, and the ability to reason, but left others intact and capable of functioning. They asked a number of questions which indicated their interest and desire to learn about the nature of the disease and the problems faced by the family.

The only available place to meet in the nursing home was a very small library. In the center of the library was a table, and on the table was a wire cage inhabited by a parrot. Fortunately, the bird did not enter into our conversation, but its activities did distract one student. Other than that, I considered the meeting very satisfactory. The students showed interest, observed closely, and some took notes. As I recall, there were two young women in the group who asked more questions, talked more, and took more notes than the three young men combined.

Before the meeting, I was in doubt as to how to introduce the students to Bess because I had no idea how she would respond. I decided to introduce them as my friends, who had come for a visit and wanted to see and talk with her, also. She smiled and greeted them graciously, responded well to their questions and showed no embarrassment when she could not remember. When they left, she was in good spirits, smiled, and asked them to come again. Except for her loss of memory, she was more like her old self than usual.

Before we met Bess, one student had asked me what kind of questions they should ask. I replied that there was no limit to the type of questions they might ask, although I had no idea what her responses would be. They asked a number of questions to which the answer required memory. She could not remember how many children we had, or whether our child was a boy or a girl. She did not remember from what college I had retired, or from what state we had moved to Georgia, or where we lived. When someone asked for her telephone number, she responded immediately and correctly. That was a surprise to me, for she had not been able to remember that number for more than a year. She looked at me, smiled, and said, "I bet you thought I didn't know that." The students soon discovered that, despite her loss of memory, she still had an active sense of humor.

The second meeting occurred during the period after I had withdrawn Bess from the first nursing home and four days after I had brought her home from the clinic. Although her response to the students and to their questions was not negative, it was not as positive as it had been the year before. There was less evidence of the friendliness and humor that had been so obvious in the first meeting. She didn't say, "I am happy to meet you," nor did she say, "Come to see us again," but even in her advanced condition, there were a few smiles and faint evidences of humor. She responded as best she could to questions, but there were no voluntary statements from her. She was an entirely different person from the one the first group of students had seen.

Since she could not walk without assistance, the care person remained with her. My daughter was also there, and the students directed a number of questions to her and to the care person. As a whole, I thought the students showed more intense interest in Bess and her condition than did those in the meeting the year before. All of them were kind and considerate. When one of the young ladies asked Bess if she liked to cook, she said, "Yes," but when asked what she liked to cook, she had no answer.

After about thirty minutes with Bess, I took the students to another room. This was completely different than the approach

I took the previous year, when I had met with the students first. I discovered that having seen Bess first, their interest in my problems was increased. They were more concerned with my problems as a caregiver than the previous group had been. "How do you manage to hold up under the emotional and physical burdens?" "Do you ever lose your temper?" "Do you ever become depressed?" "What are your greatest needs as a caregiver?" "Why did you withdraw her from the nursing home?" My daughter, Estelle, had gone with us, and they had an opportunity to ask her some questions about its effect on her. We had a more interesting and in-depth discussion about the problems of the caregiver than in the first meeting. I explained the importance of the support group as a source of moral support and talked about my activities to cope with both old age and Alzheimer's. When I mentioned my efforts to write a book and explain its nature, I struck a responsive chord. All expressed an interest in reading it. A few days later, I received a letter from one of the young ladies in the group thanking me for having the meeting in my home, expressing her concern for me as a caregiver, and asking me to notify her when the book had been published. I have taken so long to finish it, I fear she has forgotten. Her letter was a mark of kindness and a spark of happiness to me, such as I had never received from a doctor. I felt that she, a future doctor, had gotten the message of the Alzheimer's Awareness Program. I hope she will be able to convey her feeling to caregivers who may come into her office during her future medical career.

Each student is required by Dr. Mirra to write an evaluation of his or her experience, and the response has always been highly positive. Dr. Mirra then writes a letter of thanks to each caregiver who participates, including comments from the students who took part.

One Family Caregiver's Response

As for me, I was happy to be part of this innovative medical education program. Having spent 40 years as a teacher, I enjoyed meeting the young medical students and trying to give them a realistic, firsthand view of how it is for an elderly couple to be caught up in this kind of cruel and hopeless situation. I hope this short personal experience will help to make them a little more aware of what Alzheimer's disease can do to both its victims and their caregivers. It left me with the feeling that perhaps I had made a small contribution to a greater awareness of Alzheimer's among a few future doctors who will be practicing medicine in the next century when, unless we find a cure, it may be the disease of the century among the elderly.

The Alzheimer's Awareness Program is giving a few young medical students a short, but rare and vivid, personal experience with the problems associated with this mysterious and dreaded disease. I am confident that those who participate in this program will store that experience in their memories and never forget it. I hope that someday in the future, when the first victim of Alzheimer's disease is brought into the office by a caregiver, the doctor will recall this experience and find it helpful in treating both the patient and the caregiver.

Other Innovative Educational Programs

THE PATIENT-FOR-A-DAY PROGRAM

The patient-for-a-day program is probably one of the most interesting educational programs currently being tried in various institutions.

This program, unlike the Emory Alzheimer's program, is not aimed at any particular disease, but at physician-patient relationships and attitudes in general. One of the most universal complaints against doctors is the lack of compassion for

126

patients. Doctors don't know what it is like to be a patient nor what a patient experiences. In an effort to overcome this doctor/patient distance, a few medical schools are introducing into the medical training of their students some new educational techniques which are different from those in use at the Emory University Medical School's Alzheimer's Awareness Program. One is the role-playing technique by students, wherein students play the role of a patient for a day, to see and feel the anguish which the patient feels. A male student may be disguised as a widower recovering from a broken hip, who uses a walker and who can barely hear. A female student may play the role of an elderly widow suffering from diabetes, arthritis, and congestive heart failure, who can barely see. The hospital staff treats them as if they were real patients. This technique is in use at Hunterdon Medical Center at Fremington, New Jersey.

ASSUMING A FABRICATED ILLNESS

At the Long Beach Memorial Medical Center in Long Beach, California, residents in family care are asked to assume a fabricated illness, or illnesses, for a one-night stay in the hospital —incognito— and the staff treats them as real patients. A person may spend a sleepless night in a room with a patient who groans all night, may hear the continuous beeping of a heart monitor, and may see nurses coming in and out all night.

OTHER APPROACHES

At the Uniformed Services University of the Health Sciences at Bethesda, Maryland, the entire entering class is issued bedpans and told to use them. This may result in some self-conscious and silly experiences. Some schools have engaged actors to portray ornery and uncooperative patients, whom the students are asked to interview.

The purpose of such techniques is to help future doctors understand what patients feel, to have compassion for them, and to relate to them. Such experiences may help doctors to deal with some of the painful emotional and moral issues which often arise in the practice of medicine. There is, of course, some disagreement among doctors about these techniques. Some fear it may threaten the objectivity of the practicing physician. It is vitally important that objectivity be preserved, but it certainly helps to have a little compassion and empathy to go along with it. These techniques are in the early stages of development, but there is some evidence that they may leave some lasting memories, which will help doctors in dealing with patients. For example, one doctor has reported that the role he played as a student patient made him feel silly and self-conscious, but it later helped him refrain from blowing his top when dealing with a patient who had suffered a brain injury and was ornery and verbally abusive, throwing bedpans and pulling out catheters. He said, "I recognized that the patient was scared to death, confused, and had lost a great deal of his dignity. That made me able to deal with him." ⚭

THINKING THE UNTHINKABLE

Death by Euthanasia

Someone has said that we are a "death-denying" society. It is not so much that we deny death, but rather, that we fail to think realistically about it and prepare for it before it is upon us. Many religious people think of death as God's work and believe Man has no right to do anything about it, except to relieve pain. The marvels of modern medical science—the respirator, the feeding tube, and life-sustaining drugs—have made it possible to preserve the life of an ill person almost indefinitely. We are increasingly using those and other marvels of medical science for the purpose of prolonging life as long as possible when, in fact, we may be prolonging death and suffering. In our hospitals and nursing homes, human beings are making life- and-death decisions every day.

Journalist Ellen Goodman wrote, "Every year, two million Americans die, 85% of them in institutions, such as hospitals and nursing homes. Of those, 80% involve a decision by someone to do or not to do something." That something might be to insert or withdraw a feeding tube or respirator; it might be not to resuscitate an Alzheimer's patient; it might be the decision of a doctor to administer a lethal dose of morphine to end the unbearable suffering of a patient; or it might be the decision of a patient not to have another operation which might extend his or her life for only a few months.

During the last two decades, some highly publicized and controversial cases involving the withdrawal of the respirator, the feeding tube, and assisted suicide have opened our minds and made us more aware of the medical, moral, and legal dilemmas involved in such actions. The most prominent of those cases involved Karen Quinlan, Nancy Cruzan, and Janet Adkins, who committed suicide by using a machine made by a doctor. More recently, another doctor in New York has admitted assisting a patient to commit suicide. Neither doctor has been prosecuted. We have no way of knowing how many people have been helped to take their own lives, nor do we know how many doctors have resorted to euthanasia, sometimes called "mercy killing," to end the unbearable suffering of a patient.

Euthanasia and Assisted Suicide

Euthanasia, which comes from Greek words meaning "good or easy death," is often called "mercy killing"—intentional termination of life to end the intolerable suffering of a patient. Although both lead to death, it is common to draw a distinction between active euthanasia and passive euthanasia. Active euthanasia is taking some action with the intention of terminating the life of an individual, whereas an example of passive euthanasia would be withholding the feeding tube or the respirator, allowing the disease to run its course and the patient to die a natural death.

A type of euthanasia is practiced in Holland, but it has never been legalized by an act of the Dutch parliament. The Dutch government authorized a State Commission on Euthanasia to study the issue, and its report favored allowing physicians to perform euthanasia under certain conditions and in accordance with a number of specific safeguards. The Dutch Supreme Court has ruled that performing euthanasia is no longer to be prosecuted if performed in compliance with those safeguards.

Those safeguards are: "The patient's medical situation must be intolerable, with no prospect of improvement. The patient must be rational and must voluntarily and repeatedly request euthanasia of the physician. The patient must be fully informed. There must be no other means of relieving the suffering, and two physicians must concur in the request." [9]

Since euthanasia has been more widely discussed in the United States in recent years, there is some evidence that it is becoming more favorably accepted by the people. When the Roper Poll in 1988 asked if a physician should be allowed to end the life of a terminally ill person at the patient's request, 58 percent said Yes, 27 percent said No, and 10 percent were undecided. The *Atlanta Journal-Constitution's* Southern Poll, taken in July, 1989, discovered the following from the 1,405 Southern respondents: 54 percent viewed favorably mercy killing to end the life of a terminally ill person at the patient's request; 59 percent believed that a person with an incurable disease has a moral right to end his life; and 60 percent believed that a person suffering great pain, with no hope of improvement, had the same right to take his or her own life.

What is the difference between Dutch voluntary euthanasia and assisted suicide? In voluntary euthanasia, the doctor himself performs the act which causes death; whereas, in assisted suicide, the doctor prepares the substance or the instrument of death, instructs the patient how to use it, and the patient commits the act causing death.

[9] Robert M. Baird and Stuart E. Rosenbaum, *Euthanasia, The Moral Issues*, p. 175.

The most publicized case of assisted suicide was that of Janet Adkins, a 54-year-old woman who, after being diagnosed as having Alzheimer's disease, took her life by using a suicide machine built by Jack Kevorkian, M.D. With the approval of her family, she chose to take her life, rather than suffer the eventual effects of this cruel disease. Following his instructions, she operated the machine which ended her life without his assistance. He defended his action by saying, "If there is a primal natural right, it is self-determination." "As people live longer, we increasingly face chronic, sometimes debilitating, illness. What is important is having the choice to end one's own life, at will and with dignity."

Position of the American Medical Association

The traditional role of the physician going back to ancient Greece has been to heal illness, to preserve life, and not, under any circumstance, to kill. That tradition is well-expressed in a declaration of the American Medical Association:

"The intentional termination of the life of one human being by another—mercy killing—is contrary to that for which the medical profession stands and is contrary to the policy of the American Medical Association. The cessation of extraordinary means to prolong the life of the body, when there is irrefutable evidence that biological death is imminent is the decision of the patient and/or his immediate family. The advice and judgment of the physician should be freely available to the patient and/or his immediate family."

Three important points should be noted in that statement. No doctor should intentionally terminate the life of a patient for any reason. It is permissible, however, when there is irrefutable evidence that biological death is imminent, to cease the use of extraordinary means of preserving life, despite the fact that such action might hasten the death of the patient. That decision lies in the hands of the patient and/or the family. Finally, the advice and judgment of the physician should be freely available to the patient and/or the family.

There is evidence that doctors are becoming more sensitive to the desires of a dying patient. A recent survey found that 80 percent of U.S. physicians favor withdrawing life-support systems from hopelessly ill or irreversibly comatose patients if the patient or the family request it. Dr. James Sammons, Executive Vice President of the American Medical Association, has said: "From the day they enter medical school, physicians are taught to cherish and preserve life. However, there comes the time with the terminally ill or irreversibly comatose patient that the physician must step back, at the patient's or the family's request, and allow the patient to die with dignity." He went on to say, "While physicians should never directly cause death, they must always act in the best interest of their patients, and that sometimes includes allowing them to die."

Some physicians, however, in addition to Dr. Kevorkian, are willing to go further and assist a patient to commit suicide. A physician in New York reported in the *New England Journal of Medicine* that he had prescribed sleeping pills to assist a patient to commit suicide. In Atlanta some years ago, he said, "There comes a point where the patient's comfort takes precedence over the length of his life." There is no doubt that the great majority of American physicians would reject active euthanasia. A large number, however, perhaps even a majority, would favor withholding or withdrawing life-sustaining devices if requested by the patient or the family and some would assist in suicide.

The publication of a startling how-to book, or suicide manual, renewed the controversy and thinking about assisted suicide. *Final Exit,* by Derek Humphrey, the founder and Executive

Director of the Hemlock Society, which sponsors euthanasia as a medical procedure, spells out in detail the substances and the procedures to be used in committing suicide or in helping another to do so. First published in April, 1991, it reached the bestseller list in August, and the original 41,000 copies were sold out. Mr. Humphrey says, "Part of good medicine is to help you get out of this life, as well as help you in... When a cure is no longer possible, and the patient seeks relief through euthanasia, the help of a physician is most appropriate." The great demand for such a manual indicates much interest in assisted suicide. Some people object to its sale on the grounds of misuse by teenagers and people who are temporarily depressed. Others say it represents a negative response to the medical profession's policy of permitting many terminally people to survive so long. Some bookstores refused to stock it, but the demand for it, as well as the lack of widespread efforts to stop its sales, are some indications of our willingness to think about the unthinkable.

What About the Living Dead?

There are many circumstances under which one may be forced to make life-or-death decisions. Let us take two examples: 1) Imagine an Alzheimer's victim who cannot, or will not, eat. To survive, she must be fed by running a tube down her throat, which might keep her physically alive for a number of years. What should we do? Should we withhold the tube and allow her to starve to death, which might require ten days or more? Or would it be more humane to euthanize her? 2) Now consider a different kind of case: A woman, a prospective mother, discovers that the fetus in her womb, if allowed to be born, will be the victim of Down's Syndrome. She faces a cruel dilemma. What should she do? Should she abort the fetus?

Should the law make it a criminal act to do so?

In our nursing homes, there are many people who are often called the "living dead." They are people whose hearts still beat, their lungs breath, their kidneys still function, and the digestive system can convert the food they are fed and provide the nourishment to keep them alive physically. Their brains, however, can no longer function to keep them alive mentally. They can no longer remember. They can no longer talk. They can no longer feed themselves. There is nothing they can do to give meaning to their lives. It is possible, in many cases, to keep them alive physically for a number of years. The question is, what sense does it make, and what purpose does it serve to keep them alive? How long can we afford it? Would it be better to turn our resources and attention to those who can find some joy in life? What should we do? What can we do? Should we try to find a legally and morally acceptable way to help them exit this life in a painless and dignified way? I have no answer. It is my purpose to stimulate thinking about these matters—"to think the unthinkable." We should not cease our efforts to extend life. We should increase our efforts to find a cure for the diseases which produce the living dead. We should put more emphasis on helping the elderly find a life of quality.

Let me speak for myself. Despite all my efforts to avoid it, I know I may sometime be among the living dead. The natural process of aging, Alzheimer's, or some other disabling disease may destroy my abilities to find meaning and a sense of worth in life. I have never contemplated suicide. I would not ask my doctor to commit an illegal act to help me end my life. If, however, I should be among the living dead, I hope that my doctor, acting under legally prescribed moral guidelines and with the consent of my family, will assist me to have a painless and dignified exit from this life, without fear of a malpractice lawsuit.

The Living Will and Durable Power of Attorney

Like most people, Bess and I seldom thought of death, and never in our long life together discussed it as an inevitable and eventual end to our relationship. We were slow to make any preparations for it, and had been married for more than 30 years before we wrote our first wills. We delayed longer on the purchase of burial plots and even longer on the writing of our living wills. It now seems unbelievable that two educated, informed, and responsible people would delay so long thinking about and making preparation for the inevitable fact of death. Without much discussion, we prepared and signed living wills. At that time, I had already begun to see some strange symptoms in Bess, but I did not visualize what was ahead and said nothing to her about those symptoms.

I quote the pertinent provisions of both my living will and the durable power of attorney:

THE LIVING WILL:

If, at any time, I should have a terminal condition, as defined and established in accordance with the procedures set forth in paragraph (10) of Code Section 31-32-2 of the Official Code of Georgia Annotated, I direct that the application of life-sustaining procedures to my body be withheld or withdrawn and that I be permitted to die;

In the absence of my ability to give directions regarding the use of such life-sustaining procedures, it is my intention that this living will shall be honored by my family and physician(s) as the final expression of my legal right to refuse medical or surgical treatment and accept the consequences from such refusal.

THE DURABLE POWER OF ATTORNEY:

"I, W.M. Grubbs, appoint Estelle Grubbs Neese as my attorney-in-fact (my agent if I am incapable of acting) to act for me, and in

136

my name, in any way I could act in person, to make any and all decisions for me concerning my personal care, medical treatment, hospitalization, and health care and to require, withhold, or withdraw any type of medical treatment or procedure, even though my death may ensue. My agent should have the same access to my medical records that I have, including the right to disclose the contents. My agent shall also have full power to make a disposition of any part or all of my body for medical purposes, authorize an autopsy of my body, and direct the disposition of my remains.

"If any agent named by me shall die, become legally disabled, incapacitated or incompetent, or resign, refuse to act, or be unavailable, I name the following as successors to such agent:"

As successor, I named my daughter Estelle, and as her successor, named in the power of attorney, my granddaughter. Fortunately, the only power named in the durable power used at Bess' death was the decision to have an autopsy.

Influenced by the celebrated and controversial Nancy Cruzan case, Congress passed a federal law, the Patient Self-Determination Act, which went into effect December 1, 1991. Its purpose is to give the patient control over medical treatment in health care facilities such as hospitals and nursing homes. It is concerned with what are called "advance directives"—living will or durable power of attorney, in which one may leave a written statement expressing his or her wishes about the use of life-sustaining devices, like the feeding tube and the respirator, in the event of life-threatening illness. Serious illness and accidents may leave one unable to communicate his or her wishes about the use of such instruments. In the absence of directives, the family and the doctor may be faced with life-and-death decisions without knowing the wishes of the patient. Every adult should be aware of the moral and legal dilemmas which may arise under such circumstances, should think seriously about his or her wishes and responsibilities, and should leave, in writing, advance instructions.

The federal law does not require patients to sign a living will nor to designate a proxy to make health care decisions for them, but it does require the agency to ask if they know about such directives, or if they have signed a living will or assigned to someone the durable power of attorney and if not, if they wish to do so.

The implementation of this law should help to make people more aware of the moral and legal dilemmas that often arise as one approaches death, and it should stimulate them to prepare advance directives about their wishes concerning their medical treatment. Every adult, while mentally able to do so, should sign a living will and/or a durable power of attorney expressing his or her wishes about the use of life-sustaining methods or other medical treatment. No adult should leave that responsibility to the family and/or doctor unless they have a clear knowledge of the person's wishes beforehand. ➼

CHAPTER XVI

THE END:
A PAINLESS, EASY, NATURAL DEATH

"I Am Tired of Living"

Bess loved life and was able to find pleasure and a sense of worth in what she did and in her relationships with other people. We had a happy marriage. She was not the type of person who would become tired of living without some profound change affecting her nature. She had a positive attitude toward life and a great sense of humor and would seldom think of death. She would never think of taking her own life, nor that of any other person.

We had been married for more than thirty years before we bought burial lots; once we had them, there was no further talk of death until we decided to have a living will written. When Bess started talking about changing our burial place, I saw it as a sign that she was thinking about death. She finally ceased talking about the burial plots, but she began to threaten suicide.

Among all her housekeeping duties, cooking had been the most meaningful and enjoyable for her. She retained a deep obsession with cooking, even after she had lost all interest in other household duties. With the onset of dementia, she lost her conception of the time to cook and would start cooking any time of day. She lost her ability to cook without burning food, but she clung to her feeling of the necessity to cook. She could no longer do needlecraft; she could no longer read, watch television, nor socialize. Cooking seemed to her the last and only meaningful thing to do.

She resented the fact that I was taking away from her the only remaining activity which she could think of doing. Most of her threats to take her life occurred in the kitchen, and my angriest moments with her were there. I am sure that she did not, in most cases, really mean to kill herself because she never attempted to do so. Her threats were an expression of her anger toward me. The only time she ever threatened to divorce me occurred in the kitchen. She actually told me that she had consulted a lawyer about it. During her first few months in the nursing home, she often threatened to commit suicide, but that finally ceased.

It was not until she had spent two years in the nursing home that she put into words her feeling about life which was out of character for her. It occurred in the interval between withdrawal from the first home and placing her in the second. She had almost recovered from the heavy sedation at the clinic and was at home with me. One morning at breakfast I asked, "How do you feel today?" She replied, "I am tired of living." I am sure she meant it and that this was a true expression of her feelings throughout her four years in nursing homes. The happiest moments of her life in the nursing home were those I spent with her. I was told by a nurse and others, "Just stay away and she will forget. Your coming to see her so often hinders her adjustment to the nursing home." But as long as she recognized me and found my visits enjoyable, I could not stay away. Only a heartless person would do that and I am not that kind of person. Based on my experience and observations in the nursing homes, that is what happens to many residents. We warehouse them and leave them to sit there in boredom and social isolation waiting for death.

Some Bad Omens

Some bad omens began to appear as far back as eighteen months before Bess died. She had pneumonia from which she had never completely recovered; she was confined to a wheelchair, and she began to have frequent respiratory failures and congestive heart failure. I had to live with the knowledge that she might die quickly and unexpectedly from the congestive heart failure. Other than those problems, she appeared to be in very good physical health. She remained very alert and was able to feed herself with little help. We spent many pleasant hours in the lobby looking at magazines, but her frequent spells of difficulty in breathing kept me aware of the danger which was ever present.

One night, about three months before her death, another puzzling and bad omen occurred. The nurse called to report that Bess had been vomiting coffee grains. That puzzled and worried me. She did not drink coffee and even if she did, she would not have ingested enough to be vomiting grains. Later that night, I was told that Bess had gone to bed and was all right. The next day I was told that what the night nurse had seen was probably dried blood. That concerned me because it was apparently the result of internal bleeding which could be serious. A check of her stool, however, showed no evidence of such a problem. That eased my concern somewhat, but it did not answer the major question: Where did that blood come from?

About two months later, my daughter, Estelle, and I took Bess to the hospital for a blood transfusion and a G.I. series in an effort to find the source of the bleeding. It took about eight hours to have a transfusion of two pints of blood. Bess did not understand why she was there, nor what was being done for her. Since she refused to cooperate, it was very difficult to take blood samples, take her temperature, and insert the transfusion tube. If we had left her for even a minute, she would have pulled the tube out. Like a broken record, she said all day long, "I want to go home. I want to go home." There was nothing we could do or say to stop her. When we returned a few days later for the G.I. series, it took nine hours! Since we were not allowed in the X-ray room, we sat in an adjoining waiting room where we could hear her protesting loudly about everything they did. The upper G.I. was done through a series of X-ray pictures taken every thirty minutes. During the intervening time, she was brought out to be with Estelle and me. Again, all day long, she repeated over and over, "I want to go home." Estelle and I have never spent two more miserable days in our lives. We were more exhausted than Bess. I decided then that I would never again subject her to such an ordeal.

Because of her refusal to cooperate, the barium enema and the upper G.I. series produced very poor results. They did discover a hiatus hernia and diverticulitis, and concluded that the bleeding came from the latter.

"Just Sitting Here Waiting For The End"

I was encouraged by the improved color in Bess' face following the transfusion. Her hemoglobin improved, but had not reached normal at the time of her death. I was also encouraged by the fact that she was eating better and seemed more alert. My hopes soon collapsed, however, on a visit to have lunch with her. On that day I found her sitting alone, staring into space. I walked up behind her, tapped her on the shoulder, and kissed her, and I was surprised when she asked, "Where did you come from?" I did not mention home, but said, "I just walked in from the outside." I then asked "How are you today?" She replied, "It's horrible just sitting here waiting for the end." Although I tried to get her to tell me what she meant, she would or could not. She had spoken more fluently than usual. While I was surprised by her statement, I think that it was an expression of the suffering that she had experienced for several months. I believe she still had enough cognitive ability to realize that the end was not far away. She had given up hope, and was just sitting there waiting for it. That had a devastating emotional impact on me. Although I did not want her to die, I knew that death was inevitable sooner or later, and I could not help thinking what a relief it would be for her when death finally ended her suffering. To go home and leave her there alone, staring into space, waiting for death, was the hardest thing I ever did. It seemed like deserting her at a time when she needed me most. How could I do that to the woman I loved and had lived with for so long? I could not take her home, and even if I did, she would not recognize it as home. I knew that I could not stay with her day after day without risking my own mental and emotional well-being. The decision not to bring her home broke my heart. Under such circumstances, one may doubt his faith in God and ask, "Where is He? Why does he allow this kind of thing to go on? If He is the merciful, all-loving, and compassionate Being we say he is, why doesn't He end this suffering?"

On April 7, 1991, I went as usual to have lunch with Bess, found her slumped over in the wheelchair, unable to sit up or hold her head straight. She was strapped in the chair to keep from falling. I immediately inquired of the nurse if she had been heavily sedated, and was told that she was not under sedation, but she had been in that condition since morning. She seemed alert and said, "Let's go home." I wheeled her to the dining room where we had lunch. She seemed hungry and ate everything on her plate. Since she could not lift a fork to her mouth, I fed her. After lunch when we went to the lobby to look at magazines, she showed no interest. I turned the pages and pointed to pictures which I thought might interest her, but it was no use; she kept asking to go home. Since there was nothing I could do or say to entertain her or stop her from asking to go home, I left earlier than usual, and decided to return to have dinner with her later.

That evening, I found her no better, and her words were more slurred than usual, but she was hungry. As soon as her dinner tray was placed before her, she tried to get a mouthful of food with her fingers, like a little child who had not learned to use a fork and spoon. When I fed her, she ate nearly everything on her plate. I knew that something was happening to her, but it puzzled me that she was still eating well.

After dinner I returned home and called soon after to inquire about her. The nurse told me that she was still awake and was having difficulty breathing although I had not noticed her experiencing any difficulty in breathing during my visit. The nurse added that she had been given medication for the breathing, and assured me that Bess would go to sleep after the medication took effect. However, at nine-thirty, the nurse called to report that the doctor had been called and was on his way. My daughter and my grandson rushed me to the nursing home where we found Bess in a coma breathing with the aid of oxygen. It seemed she had had a stroke and the doctor offered to arrange to take her to the hospital. When I inquired if that would do any good he said, "No." I replied, "Let's not take her." He then said it was only a matter of time — it might be within hours, or two or three days. If I wished, he would give her antibiotics and other medication. I inquired again if he thought they would help.

When he again said, "No," I replied, "Let's not do it." Since I was convinced the time for her to go had come, it was useless to give her further medication. I had thought for eighteen months that she would most likely die of respiratory failure and congestive heart failure, and had requested that if she reached that condition, no effort be made to resuscitate her. Bess and I had agreed on that before she became a victim of Alzheimer's.

The nurse brought a chair to Bess's bedside for me. After watching her for a while, I reached over and touched her hand. She opened her eyes, recognized me, and reached out both hands. I leaned down, kissed her on the forehead, and she slipped back into a coma.

In the meantime, Estelle, her husband, and my granddaughter arrived. At two-thirty, they insisted that I go home and get some rest. I knew I had some difficult days ahead, but believed Bess would last through the night. At five-thirty, Estelle came to my bedroom, and said, "She passed away at four-thirty."

Following her death, a flood of emotions ran through me: grief, disappointment, guilt, regrets, and a loneliness for the one who had been a part of my life for so long. Despite these feelings, there was relief that her long suffering was over and happiness that her death had been painless and easy rather than a long and painful experience.

Among my regrets, the most difficult to bear has been that I was not with her when she died. During our long life together, when one of us left on a journey, we always hugged, kissed, and said "Good-bye." She had now gone on her final journey alone, and we had not been able to say our customary good-bye. Such a parting would have been an emotional and tearful experience, but a fitting end to our long life together.

I needed the chance to cleanse myself of the guilty feelings which had accumulated during her illness. I had lied to her as a coping device and had denied her information about the death of a sister and a brother. I was disappointed that it was not possible to tell her I was sorry at the end. Her death would have been easier for me to accept had we been able to say that final good-bye.

I have not been able to rid myself of the feeling that she may have aroused at the very moment of death and reached out for me, but I was not there. If that did happen, what a horrible feeling it must have been for her! It has left me with the thought that I failed her at the moment she needed me most. I can accept her death, but I have been unable to cope with my failure to be with her at the moment of death.

The Official Certificate Of Death

Although at least three factors contributed to her death, we will never know which was the most important, and it makes no difference now. The official death certificate read as follows: "Respiratory failure, chronic obstructive lung disease, and/or accident." Her death was quick, painless, easy, and natural, the kind of death for which we both had hoped. It brought an end to the confusing, meaningless life which she had suffered for so many years.

The Truth Revealed: The Autopsy

The autopsy stated the following: "We were indeed able to confirm the diagnosis of Alzheimer's disease in your wife, Bess. In examining sections of the brain under the microscope, we did see many neurofibrillary tangles and senile plaques which, as you know, are the hallmarks of this disease. In addition, there was prominent scarring or loss of brain cells in an area of the brain believed to be critical for memory function. This was more severe than we see in most of our Alzheimer's disease cases."

146

"This case is interesting in that, in many regions of cortex there are only moderate numbers of senile plaques and many of these are of the diffuse subtype. However, in other regions, for example, the temporal lobe, the numbers of neuritic plaques meet accepted conventional histopathological criteria for the diagnosis of Alzheimer's disease. Superimposed on these changes, however, there is significant gliosis in the entorhinal cortex. We have encountered such changes in patients with dementia, both in the presence and absence of concomitant Alzheimer's disease pathology."

The Beginning of The Rest of My Life

Bess and I had lived so long and so well together that we had become a part of each other. The other half of me, the best parts of my life, died and were buried with her. Nothing except Alzheimer's, or a similar brain-killing dementia, can wipe out the memories of our life together. As long as my memory lasts, I will not forget the joys, the sorrows, the disappointments, the failures, and the achievements we shared. She is now gone, and I face the future alone, and must find a new life of my own which is worth living in her absence. In many cases, grief from the death of a spouse is so overwhelming that it shortens the life of the surviving one, or leaves him or her with an empty, lonely, and unhappy existence. I must not allow that to happen to me.

I know that time has a healing effect on grief, but time needs help from me. People have a great potential for self-healing if they will discover and use it. Each individual must find his or her ways to assist time in the healing process. We must examine our nature, our interests, and our own physical and mental capabilities and choose the ways most suitable for us. My ways may not be your ways. As for me, I face the future with a positive attitude toward life, a young-at-heart spirit, and a desire to find something worth doing. I will not allow my physical and mental qualities to atrophy through lack of use. There is so much I want to know, so much I want to see, and so much I want to do that if I should live to be one hundred twenty, I could not know it all, see it all, nor do it all. I will not become a recluse, but will preserve my present friendships and seek new ones to escape a sense of social isolation. I will try to retain my sense of humor and find a few laughs along the way. Yes, I will cry on occasions because I miss Bess and wish that she were here to share a good life with me. I have hope and confidence that I will be able to reduce the crying and yield to it only on special occasions, and that I will find a life of fulfillment and happiness. Hope and confidence are great therapy for the bereaved.

The Alzheimer's Support Group for the Bereaved

Shortly after Bess' death, I received from the local chapter of the Alzheimer's Association the announcement of a new support group for the bereaved. Among the seven people who attended the meetings of this first group were a man who had lost a wife to Alzheimer's Disease, a woman who had lost a husband, and the remainder had lost their mothers. Two members of the chapter office shared the leadership of our discussions.

Like the caregivers support group, this new group was based on the principle of self-help and moral support for those struggling with the overwhelming grief from the loss of a loved one. All who are suffering such grief need to express their feelings, and to share them with other people. There is no better place to do it than among others who are experiencing similar feelings. Such meetings are very emotional but each member leaves with a sense of relief and some knowledge of how others are dealing with grief. ⭖

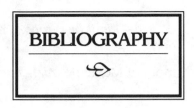

BIBLIOGRAPHY

Aronson, Miriam K., Editor, Ed. D. *Understanding Alzheimer's Disease: What It Is, How To Cope with It.* Charles Scribner's and Sons,1988.

Baird, Robert M. and Stuart E. Rosenbaum, Editors, *Euthanasia, the Moral Issues.* Prometheus Books, New York, 1989

Butler, Robert N., M.D. *Why Survive? Being Old In America* Harlers Torchbooks, New York, 1975.

Callahan, Daniel, *Setting Limits: Medical Goals in an Aging Society.* Simon & Schuster, 1987

Carroll, David L., *When Your Loved One Has Alzheimer's.* Harper and Row, New York, 1989

Cohen, Donna, Ph.D. and Eisdorfer, Carl, Ph.D., *The Loss of Self: A Family Resource for Caregivers of Alzheimer's Disease and Related Disorders.* NAL Penguin Inc., 1987

Coons, Dorothy H., Lena Metzelaar, Anne Robinson, and Beth Spencer, Editors, *A Better Life: Helping Family Members, Volunteers and Staff Improve the Quality of Life of Nursing Home Residents suffering from Alzheimer's Disease and Related Disorders.* Source for Nursing Home Literature, Columbus, Ohio. 1986

Dippel, Raye Lynne, Ph.D. and J. Thomas Hutton, M.D., Ph.D., editors, *Caring for the Alzheimer's Patient.* Prometheus Books. 1988

Doernberg, Myra, *The Stolen Mind.* Algonquin Books, Chapel Hill, N.C., 1986

Donnelly, John, Ed., *Suicide, Right or Wrong?* Prometheus Books, New York, 1990

Emory University School of Medicine, *Alzheimer's Disease,* 1988 Update

French, Carolyn J., LMSW, *Long Term Care Insurance: A Georgia Consumer's Guide*

Gerontology Research Center, National Institute on Aging, *Normal Human Aging: The Baltimore Longitudinal Study of Aging.* 1984

Gwyther, Lisa P., ACSN, *Care of Alzheimer's Patients: A Manual for Nursing Home Staff.* American Health Care Association, 1985

Heston, Leonard L., M.D. and June White, *Dementia, A Practical Guide to Alzheimer's Disease and Related Illnesses.* W.H. Freeman and Company, 1983

Lammers, William W., *Public Policy and the Aging.* CQ Press, A Division of the Congressional Quarterly. 1983

Mace, Nancy L., and Peter V. Rabins, M.D. *The 36-Hour Day.* The Johns Hopkins University Press, 1982

Manning, Doug, *When Love Gets Tough; The Nursing Home Decision* Insight Books

Monk, Abraham, Editor, *The Age of Aging,* Prometheus Books, 1979

National Geographic Society, *The Incredible Machine (The Human Body).* 1986

National Geographic, *Our Immune System, The Wars Within,* June 1986

National Institute on Aging, *Special Report on Aging,* 1987.

Office of Technology Assessment, *Losing A Million Minds, Confronting the Tragedy of Alzheimer's and Other Dementias.* U.S. Government Document, 1987

Reader's Digest Association, Inc., *The ABC's of the Human Body*, 1987

Restak, Richard M., M.D. *The Mind*, Bantam Books, 1988

Scully, Thomas, M.D., and Celia Scully, *Playing God*, Simon and Schuster, 1987

Torstar Books, *The Brain*, 1984

Zgola, Jitka M., *Doing Things, A Guide to Programming Activities for Persons with Alzheimer's Disease and Related Disorders*, Johns Hopkins University Press, 1987

OTHER RESOURCES FROM ELDER BOOKS

Gone Without A Trace by Marianne Caldwell

Stella Dickerman, an accomplished artist and weaver, vanished mysteriously on September 13, 1991, two years after the onset of Alzheimer's disease. *Gone Without A Trace* is the gripping personal story of her daughter's quest for answers during the long search odyssey which ensued. A first-of-its-kind, *Gone Without A Trace* provides unique insight into the profound pain endured by the families of missing persons, and offers sensitive guidance on how to comfort them. **$10.95**

Surviving Alzheimer's: A Guide for Families
by Florian Raymond

Easily digestible, this book is a treasure house of practical tips, ideas and survival strategies for the busy caregiver. It describes how to renew and restore yourself during the ups and downs of caregiving, and shows you how to take care of yourself as well as your family member. **$10.95**

Failure-Free Activities for the Alzheimer's Patient
by Carmel Sheridan

This award-winning book describes hundreds of simple, non-threatening activities which are suitable for persons with Alzheimer's disease. The author describes how to focus on the abilities that remain rather than the patient's deficits and shows how to create activities which capitalize on existing strengths. **$10.95**

Reminiscence: Uncovering A Lifetime of Memories
by Carmel Sheridan

Reminiscing is one of the most powerful healing activities for people with Alzheimer's disease. This book explains the simple techniques involved in stimulating memories. It outlines themes to explore, as well as hundreds of meaningful activities involving reminiscence.

$12.95

ORDER FORM

Send To:

Elder Books   Post Office Box 490   Forest Knolls CA 94933
PH: 1 800 909 COPE (2673)   FAX: 415 488-4720

Please send me:

Qty.		Price/copy	Totals
____	*In Sickness & in Health*	@ $12.95	$____.__
____	*Show Me the Way to Go Home*	@ $10.95	$____.__
____	*Gone Without A Trace*	@ $10.95	$____.__
____	*Surviving Alzheimer's: A Guide for Families*	@ $10.95	$____.__
____	*Failure-Free Activities*	@ $10.95	$____.__
____	*Reminiscence*	@ $12.95	$____.__

Total for books . . . . $____.__
Total sales tax . . . . $____.__
Total shipping . . . . $____.__
Amount enclosed . . . . $____.__

Shipping: $2.50 for first book, $1.25 for each additional book; California residents, please add 8.25% sales tax.

Name

Address

City   State   Zip